Group Treatment for Substance Abuse

A STAGES-OF-CHANGE THERAPY MANUAL

Mary Marden Velasquez

Gaylyn Gaddy Maurer

Cathy Crouch

Carlo C. DiClemente

Foreword by William R. Miller

THE GUILFORD PRESS
New York   London

© 2001 The Guilford Press
A Division of Guilford Publications, Inc.
72 Spring Street, New York, NY 10012
www.guilford.com

Printed in the United States of America

This book is printed on acid-free paper.

Last digit is print number: 9 8 7 6 5 4 3 2

Library of Congress Cataloging-in-Publication Data

Group treatment for substance abuse : a stages-of-change therapy manual / Mary Marden
  Velasquez . . . [et al.] ; foreword by William R. Miller.
     p. cm.
  Includes bibliographical references and index.
  ISBN 1-57230-625-4 (pbk.)
  1. Substance abuse—Treatment. 2. Group psychotherapy. I. Velasquez, Mary Marden.
RC564 .G76 2001
616.86′0651—dc21

2001031358

About the Authors

Mary Marden Velasquez, PhD, is Associate Professor in the Department of Family Practice and Community Medicine at the University of Texas–Houston Medical School. Dr. Velasquez's background and training are in the areas of clinical psychology, health psychology, and public health. For the past 15 years, she has been involved in the conceptualization, design, and implementation of many studies using the transtheoretical model of behavior change. Dr. Velasquez's recent work has included development of stage-based interventions in the areas of HIV prevention, respiratory health, prenatal health, alcohol abuse, smoking cessation, and the prevention of fetal alcohol syndrome.

Gaylyn Gaddy Maurer, MA, has worked with the transtheoretical model for the past 10 years. She is currently a faculty member with the Addiction Research and Treatment Division of the University of Colorado Health Sciences Center. She has worked in the substance abuse field in both research and clinical settings with a variety of populations, including veterans, felony probationers, the dually diagnosed homeless, women at risk for alcohol-exposed pregnancies, and adolescents in residential treatment and day treatment.

Cathy Crouch, MSW, is Director of Programs with the SEARCH Homeless Project in Houston, Texas. She has extensive management experience in corporate, academic, and social service settings. Ms. Crouch is a licensed clinical social worker who has worked in research institutions, as well as inpatient and outpatient treatment facilities. She has published in the area of mental illness and substance abuse among the homeless.

Carlo C. DiClemente, PhD, is Professor and Chair of the Department of Psychology at the University of Maryland, Baltimore County. Dr. DiClemente is the codeveloper, with Dr. James Prochaska, of the transtheoretical model of behavior change. Over the past 20 years, he has written numerous scientific articles, books, and book chapters examining the process of human behavior change and the application of this model to a variety of behaviors. Dr. DiClemente has directed an outpatient alcoholism treatment program based on the transtheoretical model and served as a consultant to the National Institute on Drug Abuse, the National Institute on Alcohol Abuse and Alcoholism, the Center for Substance Abuse Treatment, and both private and public treatment programs. Dr. DiClemente is a coauthor of a self-help book based on this model of change, *Changing for Good,* and several professional books applying the model to addictive and health behaviors. He has presented this model in training workshops in the United States, Canada, Great Britain, Europe, Mexico, and New Zealand.

Acknowledgments

I, Mary Velasquez, would like to thank my family—Jerry, Keith, and Daniel—for their support and encouragement of this work. Many others have provided invaluable critiques and creative ideas, notably Kirk von Sternberg, Danielle SoRelle-Miner, and Dr. Joseph Carbonari. Dr. Jan Groff has been a source of inspiration and a truly supportive friend and colleague. Studies such as Project MATCH and Positive Choices (funded by the National Institute on Alcohol Abuse and Alcoholism), Smoke-Free Families (funded by the Robert Wood Johnson Foundation), and Project CHOICES (funded by the Centers for Disease Control and Prevention) have contributed to the body of knowledge contained in this manual. Central to these studies, of course, are the fine investigative teams that helped shape my thoughts about substance abuse and behavior change. In particular, Drs. Jeffrey Parsons, Pat Mullen, Louise Floyd, Karen Ingersoll, and Mark Sobell have willingly shared their rich and varied expertise on our mutual projects.

A great deal of credit also goes to Drs. William Miller and Stephen Rollnick, and the incredibly talented Motivational Interviewing Network of Trainers (fondly known as "Minties"). For the last several years, I have had the honor of participating in this network and experiencing "live" some of the finest thinking and inquisitive minds in the field. In particular, Jacki Hecht, Angelica Thevos, and David Rosengren have provided insight and encouraged me through the high and low times in the development of this manual.

I cannot think of any more important thanks than those that Gaylyn, Cathy, and I extend to our coauthor, Dr. Carlo DiClemente. Carlo has been a role model extraordinaire. We have been inspired by his talent and creativity, impressed (and exhausted) by his energy and productivity, and, most importantly, awed by his commitment to the field and his unwavering integrity. It is with Carlo's encouragement and direction that we have come to appreciate the important connection between research and clinical work in substance abuse, and the value of developing meaningful ways to bridge the two.

I, Gaylyn Maurer, thank my loving and patient husband, Joseph, without whose support and willingness to endure many lonely, late nights and hours caring for our son, Nicholas, I could not have invested the time needed to help complete this work.

I, Cathy Crouch, would like to acknowledge first the role that SEARCH Homeless Project, its staff, and clients have played in the development of this manual. Don Hall provided many helpful ideas about chapters to be included in the book. Irene Grosdanis, while a graduate student, spent almost a year doing the background research for the original version. John Cleveland has conducted Action Maintenance Groups over the past year and a half, providing valuable feedback.

I am especially appreciative to Don Hennigan, whose love and encouragement sustained me while working on this project. Last, I owe an intellectual debt to Dr. Fernando Flores, of Business Design Associates, to whom I dedicate this work. Through his research in linguistic theory, continental philosophy, and management theory, he has helped shape my way of constructing the world.

I, Carlo DiClemente, would like to thank the many colleagues at the Texas Research Institute of Mental Sciences (TRIMS) and, in particular, the late Dr. Jack Gordon, who encouraged the clinical application of the transtheoretical model. Colleagues and staff who pioneered efforts to develop the Alcoholism Treatment Clinic at TRIMS contributed much to the thinking that underlies the clinical wisdom reflected in this book. The many colleagues, graduate students, and workshop participants who asked good questions, shared clinical experiences, and offered ideas were particularly helpful in shaping the clinical application of concepts. They are too many to name but Carlo is grateful to each and every one of them. Coauthors Mary, Gaylyn, and Cathy, deserve most of the credit for this work. Their dedication, energy, vision, and hard work have been an inspiration. Finally, I want especially to thank my wife, Lyn, and delightful daughters, Cara and Anna, for their love and support through all of the travel, absences, and work to do the research and attend the meetings that are part of the process of bringing ideas to practice.

Finally, our sincere thanks go to Barbara Watkins, our editor at The Guilford Press, for her insight and wisdom. Barbara's understanding of the transtheoretical model and her incisive questions helped clarify our ideas. Many times, she saw better than we did how the parts formed a whole. She has been a true partner in helping us bring this work to press.

Foreword

It would be difficult to find an innovation that has had a more substantial impact on addiction treatment during the past 30 years than the transtheoretical model of behavior change (TTM). Starting from basic research with tobacco smokers, the TTM quickly spread to address alcohol and other drug problems, and indeed far beyond the addiction field to broad applications in psychotherapy, health care, and organizational settings. Among addiction treatment professionals, the TTM stages of change are now nearly as familiar as the 12 steps of Alcoholics Anonymous (AA).

In particular, thinking about substance use disorders in the United States has undergone radical change since the 1960s, and the TTM has played a significant role in that transition to new models. Smoking, drinking, drug use, and gambling—once seen as very distinct, even unrelated phenomena—have come to be seen as "addictive behaviors" that are more similar than different. The common stages, processes, and levels of change described in TTM have supported this view of addictive behaviors as similar and interrelated.

TTM work has also done much to encourage behavioral health professionals to address addictive behaviors, which were once regarded in the United States as the exclusive province of recovering paraprofessional addiction counselors. People with substance use disorders often present with a plethora of other psychological, health, and social problems, some of which are understandably of greater concern to the client than substance use itself. TTM naturally encourages one to think of addictive behavior as *behavior*, responsive to a wide variety of influences and interventions.

Addiction counseling in the United States during the 1960s was also mired in a misguided application of the psychodynamic concept of defense mechanisms, particularly denial. Clients who were "not ready" for what addiction professionals had to offer were often blamed or dismissed or confronted for their lack of behavior change. TTM provides a very different way of thinking about motivation for change. Contemplation of, preparation for, and initiation of action are seen as natural, sequential steps toward stable change. Rather than blaming clients for being unmotivated, TTM encourages one to understand the client's present stage of change, and to provide counseling that is appropriate to his or her current level of readiness. Enhancing motivation for change thus becomes part of the counselor's job, and not the sole responsibility of the client.

I find it gratifying and a bit amusing that when I write and speak now about the U.S. disease model and confrontation, recently trained professional audiences are sometimes incredulous that addiction treatment was ever conceptualized and practiced in such a manner. Indeed, from the retrospection of the maintenance stage, people often find amazement and humor in recalling a life of precontemplation. In the U.S. addiction field, the 1960s might be characterized as the precontemplation stage, the 1970s as contemplation, the 1980s as preparation, and the 1990s as action in the transition to a new paradigm for understanding and treating addictions. If that is so, then the 21st century poses the new challenges of maintenance and relapse prevention.

In that regard, this is a timely volume. Models that are understood at first as simple tend to become more complex over time. People who find their way into AA may start out with a born-again zeal and a black-and-white absolutism that serves them during early sobriety. Over the years, they may develop a more subtle and deeper understanding of the program of AA and its 12 steps. Many addiction professionals can now name and briefly explain the TTM stages of change. Less familiar but just as central to TTM are the *processes* of change. Too often, applications of TTM are oversimplified. "Stage-matched" interventions may be reduced to identifying a client's stage of change, and pulling off the shelf the appropriate instructions corresponding to that stage. If only it were so simple.

What is refreshingly different about this new clinical resource from Mary Marden Velasquez and her colleagues is its explication of the 10 TTM processes of change, which in effect suggest a menu of strategies from which to design individualized change plans. The focus of this book is on substance use, but like motivational interviewing, the processes are applicable well beyond addiction treatment. The book is structured to guide a comprehensive 29-session group treatment, but in fact, the methods and exercises can be useful in group or individual counseling and are applicable in shorter or longer courses of treatment. This highly structured outline will be a useful starting point for counselors starting out with TTM and group treatment. More experienced clinicians may prefer to apply the concepts and strategies in a more flexible manner. What this book offers overall is a consistent theoretical framework for deciding what to do when, in helping people move through the stages of change.

The authors also incorporate motivational interviewing as a clinical style to be used throughout the course of treatment. This has been our experience as well, that the client-centered style originally described by Carl Rogers and his colleagues serves us well and, indeed, improves client outcomes when applied throughout treatment. This is in contrast to the view that one uses the clinical style of motivational interviewing until the client is past the contemplation stage, and then shifts into a directive instructional style. It is a clinical challenge to provide directive cognitive-behavioral treatment while actively practicing accurate empathy, genuineness, and unconditional positive regard. It is also how I believe addiction treatment should be done.

This book is a beginning. The treatment approach that it describes is well specified and now needs to be tested for its impact on client outcomes. Beyond documenting the effectiveness of this approach, research will be warranted to study the change processes that underlie any observed effects. Do clients undergoing this treatment in fact show greater or more rapid progress through the stages of change? Are such changes predictive of stable behavior change? Is the treatment particularly helpful for people who enter treatment at certain stages of change? How does the impact of the full 29-session treatment compare with that of briefer forms, or of the same basic approach applied flexibly in order to individualize treatment? Can clients enter the group at any point in the cycle, or is it important to "work the program" from the beginning, in its prescribed order? To what extent do therapists differ in their success in using this treatment?

In the meantime, this therapist manual represents a sensible next step in the translation of TTM theory and research into a substance use treatment approach. Others have pursued a stage-matching strategy, but this approach uses TTM theory itself to mobilize the very processes of change that people use in their daily lives. That application of not just the stages, but the *processes* of change, is one of the things that I like most about this book, and that represents part of its distinctive contribution to the addiction treatment field.

WILLIAM R. MILLER, PhD
Distinguished Professor of Psychology and Psychiatry
The University of New Mexico

Contents

Introduction   1

PART I. HOW TO HELP PEOPLE CHANGE

Chapter 1. How People Change: The Transtheoretical Model   7
An Overview of the Model, 7
Doing the Right Thing at the Right Time, 9
Moving through the Stages of Change, 11
How the Processes Facilitate Movement through the Stages, 13
The Differences between Processes of Change and Techniques, 16
Adapting This Manual to Your Needs, 16

Chapter 2. Strategies for Facilitating Change   17
A Motivational Approach, 17
Principles of Motivational Interviewing, 18
Using Motivational Interviewing to Enhance Change Process Use, 19
Motivational Strategies, 20
Overview of Techniques, 21

Chapter 3. Putting It All Together: Setting Up and Carrying Out the Intervention   27
Overview of This Treatment, 27
Who Should Conduct This Treatment, 28
In What Settings Is This Treatment Appropriate?, 28
Suggested Group Size, Frequency of Sessions, and Session Length, 29
Intake Screening and Assessment, 29
Session Format, 32
Brief Refresher on Group Work, 33
Conclusion, 35

PART II. THINKING ABOUT CHANGING SUBSTANCE USE

P/C/P Sequence: Precontemplation–Contemplation–Preparation

P/C/P Session 1: The Stages of Change   39
Change Process Objective: Consciousness Raising

P/C/P Session 2: A Day in the Life   47
Change Process Objective: Consciousness Raising

P/C/P Session 3: Physiological Effects of Alcohol   52
Change Process Objective: Consciousness Raising

P/C/P Session 4: Physiological Effects of Drugs   61
Change Process Objective: Consciousness Raising

P/C/P Session 5: Expectations   70
Change Process Objective: Consciousness Raising

P/C/P Session 6: Expressions of Concern   75
Change Process Objectives: Self-Reevaluation, Dramatic Relief

P/C/P Session 7: Values   80
Change Process Objective: Self-Reevaluation

P/C/P Session 8: Pros and Cons   84
Change Process Objective: Decisional Balance

P/C/P Session 9: Relationships   91
Change Process Objective: Environmental Reevaluation

P/C/P Session 10: Roles   97
Change Process Objective: Environmental Reevaluation

P/C/P Session 11: Confidence and Temptation   102
Change Process Objective: Self-Efficacy

P/C/P Session 12: Problem Solving   108
Change Process Objective: Self-Efficacy

P/C/P Session 13: Setting a Goal and Preparing to Change   113
Change Process Objective: Self-Liberation

P/C/P Session 14: Review and Termination   119

PART III. MAKING CHANGES IN SUBSTANCE USE

A/M Sequence: Action–Maintenance

A/M Session 1: The Stages of Change   127
Change Process Objective: Consciousness Raising

A/M Session 2: Identifying "Triggers"   135
Change Process Objective: Stimulus Control

A/M Session 3: Managing Stress   140
Change Process Objective: Counterconditioning

A/M Session 4: Rewarding My Successes   146
Change Process Objective: Reinforcement Management

Contents

A/M Session 5: Effective Communication   151
Change Process Objectives: Counterconditioning, Reinforcement Management

A/M Session 6: Effective Refusals   156
Change Process Objectives: Counterconditioning, Reinforcement Management

A/M Session 7: Managing Criticism   161
Change Process Objectives: Counterconditioning, Reinforcement Management

A/M Session 8: Managing Thoughts   166
Change Process Objectives: Stimulus Control, Counterconditioning,
Reinforcement Management

A/M Session 9: Managing Cravings and Urges   172
Change Process Objectives: Stimulus Control, Counterconditioning,
Reinforcement Management

A/M Session 10: New Ways to Enjoy Life   177
Change Process Objectives: Stimulus Control, Counterconditioning,
Reinforcement Management

A/M Session 11: Developing an Action Plan   182
Change Process Objective: Self-Liberation

A/M Session 12: Recommitting after a Slip   189
Change Process Objective: Self-Liberation

A/M Session 13: Social Support   194
Change Process Objective: Helping Relationships

A/M Session 14: Identifying Needs and Resources   199
Change Process Objective: Social Liberation

A/M Session 15: Review and Termination   206
Change Process Objectives: Self-Efficacy, Reinforcement Management

Appendix. Professional Contacts and Suggested Resources   211

References   213

Index   217

Group Treatment for Substance Abuse

Introduction

This manual is written for professionals who work with substance-abusing clients. It offers treatment strategies based on the transtheoretical model (TTM) of behavior change (Prochaska & DiClemente, 1984). The TTM offers an integrative framework for understanding, measuring, and intervening in behavior change. In this model, change is seen as a progression through a series of five stages, from an initial "precontemplation" stage, where a client is not thinking of change, to contemplation, preparation, action, on to a fifth "maintenance" stage in which the client works to maintain long-term change. In the TTM's approach to treatment, clinicians are trained to assess clients' readiness to change and to enhance client motivation through a series of techniques, depending on the client's state, or stage, of readiness.

This research-based model has precipitated a major shift in how professionals understand and treat at-risk behaviors. A critical aspect of this shift is the recognition that client motivation can be influenced. Prior to this, motivation was viewed as a trait that was not amenable to change. Treatment programs were "action-oriented"; that is, they were geared toward those clients who came through the door professing a readiness to change. If a client was considered "unmotivated," the clinician saw little hope for success. Clients not quite ready to change were considered inappropriate for treatment and either rejected from the program or treated with a confrontational approach designed to make them see the "error of their ways."

Recent approaches to treatment view motivation not as a trait, but rather as a dynamic state that can be influenced (Miller & Rollnick, 1991). This new approach to behavior change offers an exciting and refreshing perspective to the field. Clients are seen as being responsible for their own change and as having the inherent potential for change.

Research has shown that certain "change processes" facilitate clients' movement through the stages. Motivational approaches such as those identified by Miller and Rollnick (1991) complement the model and provide a method of facilitating change in the early stages, even with clients those who are resistant or not yet ready to change. Cognitive-behavioral and relapse prevention oriented strategies provide excellent tools for assisting later-stage clients in achieving and maintaining change; these strategies are even more effective when delivered using a motivational approach.

The TTM is currently being used by professionals around the world as a framework with which to examine and understand behavior change, and as a template to use in developing interventions (Prochaska, DiClemente, & Norcross, 1992). There is also an ever-increasing body of research on applying the model to numerous populations and behaviors (DiClemente & Prochaska, 1998; Stotts, DiClemente, Carbonari, & Mullen, 1996; Grimley, Prochaska, & Prochaska, 1997; Prochaska, Velicer, et al., 1994; Velasquez, Carbonari, & DiClemente, 1999; Velasquez, Crouch, von Sternberg, & Grosdanis, 2001). The model has been used by the National Cancer Institute in developing their smoking cessation materials; by several health behavior screening and treatment groups in developing their protocols, and is the leading model in the field of addiction treatment in Great Britain. Grants utilizing the model in a variety of targeted heath and addictive behavior changes have been funded by the National Cancer Institute, the National Institute on Alcohol Abuse and Alcoholism, the National Heart, Lung, and Blood Institute, the National Institute on Drug Abuse, the Centers for Disease Control and Prevention, the Robert Wood Johnson Foundation, and many other funding institutions. In a number of studies, the model constructs have been found to be sound, robust, and applicable to a wide range of health behavior problems.

Stage status and motivational readiness to change have predicted participation in treatment, treatment outcome, and long-term behavior change (DiClemente & Prochaska, 1998). The literature supports the usefulness of treatments using various components of the TTM in a variety of behaviors, including alcohol treatment (Project MATCH Research Group, 1997), alcohol prevention in adolescents (Werch, Pappas, Carlson, & DiClemente, 1999); smoking (Pallonen et al., 1994; Velicer & Prochaska, 1999; Stotts, DiClemente, & Mullen, in press), mammography (Rakowski et al., 1998), exercise (Marcus, Pinto, Simkin, Audrain, & Taylor, 1994), and HIV prevention (Collins, Kohler, DiClemente, & Wang, 1999). In summary, the literature supports the usefulness of TTM-based interventions in a variety of populations with numerous behaviors. In addition, many public mental health and substance abuse clinics are already using the TTM to inform their treatment programs. While few clinics formally evaluate their interventions, their reports on the use of this approach have been very positive, with both clients and clinicians expressing a great deal of enthusiasm.

The intervention in this manual is the first comprehensive substance abuse treatment program based on the TTM that systematically promotes movement through the stages by focusing on the processes of change. Through the use of specific techniques to promote process use, the likelihood that clients will progress through the change process is increased (Carbonari & DiClemente, 2000).

The impetus for this manual was an appeal from clinicians in a variety of settings for an intervention that provided specific directions and exercises for implementing a stage and process of change-based treatment. Initially, this manual was developed and piloted with substance-abusing clients in a program for the homeless. The response to the program, both from clinicians and clients, was overwhelmingly positive. It has since been implemented in many other substance abuse treatment facilities with a variety of clients. A great deal of anecdotal evidence supports the intervention described in this manual; however, it has not yet been evaluated in a randomized clinical trial. We encourage researchers to explore the efficacy of this approach and anticipate that future clinical trials will compare this intervention with others traditionally used in the field. This treatment lends itself well to such evaluation; reliable and valid measures exist to assess clients' progress through the stages of change, their use of the experiential and behavioral processes, their self-efficacy, and their decisional balance (DiClemente & Prochaska, 1998; Carbonari & DiClemente, 2000).

PURPOSE, GOALS, AND ORGANIZATION OF THIS MANUAL

This manual presents materials and instructions for conducting 29 group sessions designed to help people move through the stages of change and toward changing substance use. While we have written the manual to be used with groups, each session can easily be adapted for use in individual counseling. Conducted sequentially, the 29 sessions can be used to structure an entire program, either as a single sequence of 29 sessions or as two shorter sequences of 14 and 15 sessions, respectively. Alternatively, practitioners can pick and choose those sessions that seem most relevant to their setting and clients' stages of change.

Each session targets one or more processes of change at the stage when those processes are most critical to movement. The first sequence of 14 sessions is intended for clients in the early stages of change: precontemplation, contemplation, and preparation (P/C/P). These sessions are specifically designed to increase motivation and facilitate change in clients who (1) do not recognize they have a problem or are not motivated to change, (2) are thinking about changing, and (3) are preparing to change. The second, 15-session sequence is more action-oriented and is designed for clients in the later stages of change. These are clients who (1) are ready to make a behavior change, (2) are actively changing, and (3) are actively maintaining the changes they have already made. These latter sessions employ more traditional skills-building and relapse prevention strategies, again targeting particular change processes crucial for movement through preparation, action, and into longer-term action–maintenance (A/M).

The manual is organized into three main parts. In Part I, we explain the TTM in more detail and review the individual techniques that will be used to stimulate change processes in the sessions. We also describe the practical details of setting up and carrying out the intervention and introduce the basic session structure, which is consistent across all the sessions. In Parts II and III, we offer session-by-session instructions. Part II covers sessions titled "P/C/P" for clients in the early stages of change; Part III details sessions titled "A/M" for clients in the later stages of change. For each session, we present its rationale and content objectives, offer a list of materials required and a see-at-a-glance list of step-by-step session tasks, and explain how to carry out those tasks to accomplish the session objectives. Each session also includes handouts that may be copied directly from this book and distributed to clients. Chapter 3 provides more information on the session structure. We hope you will feel comfortable in adapting this manual to meet your particular needs.

PART I

How to Help People Change

CHAPTER 1

How People Change: The Transtheoretical Model

Change does not happen all at once. It takes time and energy. Much of the early change process takes place internally as a person weighs whether change is worth the time and effort required. The change process starts with a person who is unaware of any need for change. If there is a problem, the person probably ignores it or considers it unimportant. When the problem can no longer be ignored, he or she then considers what can be done about it. If the problem continues and grows in importance, definite plans to change are made. Once the person's mental, physical, and social forces have been gathered, he or she begins to struggle with the problem, taking action to make a change. If the person succeeds, he or she works at maintaining the new status. Sometimes, people "slip" back into the problem behavior. Often, however, they learn from their change attempts and it is easier to change the next time.

AN OVERVIEW OF THE MODEL

The transtheoretical model (TTM) sketched earlier shows how people successfully make changes in their lives. It is based on the research of Prochaska and DiClemente (1984), who found a number of characteristics common to all types of successful change in all types of circumstances. They found that change takes place over time in five *distinct stages of change*:

Precontemplation: not seeing a problem
Contemplation: seeing a problem and considering whether to act
Preparation: making concrete plans to act soon
Action: doing something to change
Maintenance: working to maintain the change

Prochaska and DiClemente (1984) also identified 10 specific *processes of change* that enable people to move from one stage to the next. They can be thought of as the engines of change. These processes of change fall into two groups. The first group, the experiential processes, focuses on internal thought processes and how a person views his or her situation. These processes are most relevant in the early stages of change. The second group, the behavioral processes, focuses on action and behavior, and is more important in the later stages of change. All of these processes are important elements in the movement through the stages and are critical in order to help people "do the right thing at the right time."

Briefly the 10 processes of change are as follows:

Experiential Processes

1. *Consciousness raising:* Clients gain knowledge about themselves and the nature of the behavior. Because clients may have been previously unaware of the negative effects of the substance use, learning more about it and its effects will help them make better-informed decisions.

2. *Dramatic relief:* A significant, often emotional experience related to the problem. Clients often become motivated to makes changes when their emotions are aroused by either external or internal stimuli.

3. *Self reevaluation:* The recognition of how a current behavior conflicts with personal values and life goals. Through use of this process, the client performs a thoughtful and emotional reappraisal of the behavior, and visualizes the kind of person he or she might be after making a positive change.

4. *Environmental reevaluation:* Recognition of the effects the behavior has upon others and the environment. Clients are often motivated by the realization that their substance use has not only negatively affected themselves but also other, external areas (such as people in their lives and the environments in which they function).

5. *Social liberation:* Recognition and creation of alternatives in the social environment that encourage behavior change. This process can also be seen as utilizing resources in the environment to alter and maintain changes in behavior. (Although this process is most often categorized with the experiential processes, it also functions in the later stages to help clients maintain change; see "How the Processes Facilitate Movement through the Stages" below.)

Behavioral Processes

1. *Stimulus control:* Avoidance or alteration of cues, so that the likelihood of engaging in the problem behavior is lessened. Clients who associate alcohol or drug use with specific environments (e.g., a bar during "happy hour") are less likely to engage in substance use if they avoid those "trigger" situations.

2. *Counterconditioning:* Substitution of healthy behaviors for unhealthy ones. In a situation where it is difficult for clients to alter or avoid tempting cues, an effective strategy is for clients to alter *their responses* to the cues. This often involves choosing

healthy alternatives (such as relaxing in a stressful situation) rather than abusing substances.

3. *Reinforcement management:* Rewarding of positive behavior changes. This can take the form of actual "rewards" or may simply be the positive consequences resulting from behaviors that prevent alcohol or drug use. When clients experience rewards following positive steps toward altering their substance using behavior, they are more likely to continue making similar changes.

4. *Self-liberation:* Belicf in onc's ability to change, and acting on that belief by making a commitment to alter behavior. Clients often demonstrate this process by committing to substance-related change goals.

5. *Helping relationships:* Relationships that provide support, caring, and acceptance to someone who is attempting to make a change. Clients who have abused substances often feel alienated and alone. By engaging in this change process, clients realize that they have a support system and are not isolated in addressing their substance use.

DOING THE RIGHT THING AT THE RIGHT TIME

Certain stages are marked by very low or high levels of change process activity, and importantly, specific processes are more salient in some stages than in others (Perz, DiClemente, & Carbonari, 1996). Also, many processes span adjacent stages, and some are used in varying degrees in multiple stages. Table 1.1 shows how the processes and stages relate.

Research has shown that certain change processes tend to "peak" during particular stages. The intervention sessions in this manual encourage specific process use as clients move through the stages of change. As such, the sessions have been ordered according to the most likely peak times for process use. For instance, in the early stages, the experiential processes (such as consciousness raising and self-reevaluation) are emphasized, while in later stages, more emphasis is placed on the behavioral processes (such as stimulus control and self-liberation).

The experiential processes of change (such as consciousness raising and self-reevaluation) are related to a client's "decisional balance." First introduced by Janis and Mann (1977), decisional balance refers to how a person weighs the pros and cons of a specific behavior. Practically speaking, it is a person's overall assessment of the positives (good things) and the negatives (less good things) of a specific behavior. Decisional balance has been found to indicate movement through the stages of change. People typically regard a problem behavior, such as substance abuse, favorably in the precontemplation and contemplation stages, and so they have little motivation to change it. By the action and maintenance stages, clients' decisional balance has shifted, and they typically regard a problem behavior as negative (Velicer, DiClemente, Prochaska, & Brandenburg, 1985), and take steps to alter that behavior accordingly. For instance, in precontemplation, the person doesn't see a problem, and must first become aware of the problem in order to address it; in other words, consciousness raising is needed. Growing awareness of a serious problem helps shift clients' "decisional balance" toward consideration of change. They then decide, "Is it worth the trouble to change?" As they

TABLE 1.1. The Right Change Process at the Right Time: What Helps Clients Move from Here to There?

Stage of change	From pre-contemplation to contemplation	From contemplation to preparation	From preparation to action	From action to maintenance	Staying in maintenance
Most relevant change processes	Consciousness raising				
	Dramatic relief				
	Self-reevaluation	Self-reevaluation			
	Environmental reevaluation	Environmental reevaluation			
	Decisional balance	Decisional balance			
		Self-efficacy	Self-efficacy	Self-efficacy	Self-efficacy
			Self-liberation	Self-liberation	Self-liberation
			Stimulus control	Stimulus control	Stimulus control
			Counter-conditioning	Counter-conditioning	Counter-conditioning
				Reinforcement management	Reinforcement management
			Helping relationships	Helping relationships	Helping relationships
		Social liberation			Social liberation

move through the stages, and the cons of the problem behavior are more salient, clients use the more action-oriented behavioral processes of change.

People can stay at any one stage for a long time. They can also cycle through the stages several times before finally reaching maintenance. A person who reaches the action stage and then fails to change returns to an earlier stage, perhaps contemplation. But that person is more likely to succeed next time because he or she can be better prepared.

A final key factor in successful change is clients' growing confidence in their ability to make the change. "Self-efficacy," a person's sense of how well he or she can succeed at change, is based on Bandura's (1977) social cognitive theory. In the TTM, self-efficacy has been evaluated by examining both a client's level of temptation to engage in a problematic behavior and his or her confidence to abstain from that behavior in the face of those temptations. Studies with alcohol-abusing and alcohol-dependent patients have shown that participants closer to the action stage of change demonstrate lower temptation to drink and higher confidence to abstain than patients in the earlier stages (DiClemente, Fairhurst, & Piotrowski, 1995). The difference between how tempted a person is to drink and his or her confidence to abstain from drinking in risky situations was shown to be a strong predictor of 3-year drinking outcomes in Project MATCH, a large alcohol treatment matching study; subjects whose confidence was higher than their temptation were significantly less likely to have returned to drinking at 3-year follow-up (Project MATCH Research Group, 1997). Included in P/C/P Session 11 is a self-test for temptation and confidence. This provides a relatively simple way of providing feedback to the clients, and it is written on an accessible level, so that the clients can reassess themselves as needed.

Table 1.1 depicts the relation of the change processes, decisional balance, and self-efficacy to the stages. As mentioned earlier, you will notice that some variables are relevant in more than one stage, and some span adjacent stages.

The balance of this chapter describes in greater detail these components of the TTM and how they work together.

MOVING THROUGH THE STAGES OF CHANGE

The stages of change represent points along the full course of changing. They are used to mark an individual's status in making change. Each stage of change is predictable, well defined, takes place in a period of time, and entails an associated set of cognitions or behaviors. As mentioned, there are five distinct stages of change: precontemplation, contemplation, preparation, action, and maintenance. In this section, we describe these stages and the processes associated with each. We also describe techniques that facilitate engagement in these processes, thus promoting movement through the stages.

Precontemplation

Precontemplation is the earliest stage of change. Individuals in precontemplation are unaware of problem behavior or they are unwilling, or discouraged, when it comes to changing it. They engage in little activity that could shift their view of problem behavior and can be rather defensive about the targeted problem behavior. Precontemplators are not convinced that the negative aspects of the problem behavior outweigh the positive. They are not considering change in the foreseeable future. An example of a precontemplator would be a man who drinks excessively but does not see his drinking as a problem, despite the fact that it may be affecting his work and his family life. In order to move ahead in the cycle of change, precontemplators need to recognize that there is a problem and increase their awareness of its negative aspects. Key change processes for people in this stage include consciousness raising, dramatic relief, self-reevaluation, environmental reevaluation, and tipping the decisional balance. Some techniques suggested in this manual to elicit these processes are psychoeducation (P/C/P Sessions 1, 3, and 4), cognitive recognition (P/C/P Sessions 5 and 6), and use of the Timeline Followback (P/C/P Session 2).

Contemplation

In the contemplation stage, the person acknowledges that he or she has a problem and begins to think seriously about solving it. Contemplators struggle to understand their problem, to see its causes, and think about possible solutions.

Contemplators, however, may be far from actually making a commitment to action. For example, a contemplator might gather a lot of information about treatment programs but not actually enroll. That is often the nature of contemplation. The individual knows where he or she wants to be, and maybe even how to get there, but is not quite ready to make a commitment.

Although many contemplators move on to the action stage, it is possible to spend years in the contemplation stage. The early sessions in this manual are designed to assist the contemplator in examining the reasons for his or her current behavior and to "tip the balance" in favor of change. The change processes most relevant to this stage include self-reevaluation, environmental reevaluation, social liberation, decisional balance, and self-efficacy. Suggested techniques to elicit these processes are values clarification (P/C/P Session 7), decision making (P/C/P Session 8), cognitive recognition (P/C/P Session 9), and role clarification (P/C/P Session 10).

Preparation

In the preparation stage, persons are ready to change in the near future. They are on the verge of taking action. People in this stage may have tried and failed to change before, yet they have often learned valuable lessons from past change attempts. Individuals in this stage of change need to develop a plan that will work for them. Then, they need to make firm commitments to follow through on the action option they choose. The change processes most appropriate for this stage are self-efficacy, self-liberation, stimulus control, counterconditioning, and helping relationships. Suggested techniques to elicit these processes are goal setting (P/C/P Session 13), framing (A/M Session 12), and problem solving (P/C/P Sessions 11 and 12).

Action

In the action stage, people most overtly modify their behavior. They stop smoking, remove all the desserts from the house, pour the last beer down the drain, or enter a treatment program. In short, they make the move and implement the plan for which they have been preparing.

Action is the most obviously busy period and the one that requires the greatest commitment of time and energy. Changes made during the action stage are more visible to others than those made during the other stages, and therefore receive the greatest recognition. The danger is that many people, including professional therapists, can erroneously equate action with change, overlooking not only the critical work that prepares people for successful action but also the equally important (and often more challenging) efforts to maintain the changes following action. Key processes that help people move forward in this stage are self-efficacy, self-liberation, stimulus control, counterconditioning, reinforcement management, and helping relationships. Suggested techniques to elicit these processes are environmental restructuring (A/M Session 2), relaxation (A/M Session 3), reinforcement (A/M Sessions 4, 5, and 7), role plays (A/M Session 6), cognitive restructuring (A/M Sessions 8, 9, and 10), and relapse prevention planning (A/M Session 11).

Maintenance

Maintenance is the final stage in the process of change. Sustaining behavior change is difficult. In the maintenance stage, the person works to consolidate the gains attained during the action stage and struggles to prevent relapse. The change process does not end with the action stage. Although traditional therapy views maintenance as a static stage, the TTM sees it as a critically important continuation that can last from as little as 6 months to as long as a lifetime. Without a strong commitment to maintenance, there will surely be relapse. Often, change is not completely established even after 6 months or so of action. This is particularly true if the environment is filled with cues that can trigger the problem behavior. We all know of cases where an individual who has stopped drinking relapses just when everyone thinks the problem is finally resolved. It is important to help individuals in this stage to practice an active and intelligent maintenance of the changes they have made. Key change processes for people in this stage include strengthening self-efficacy, self-liberation, stimulus control, counterconditioning, reinforcement management, helping relationships, and social liberation. Techniques that can elicit these processes are social and communication skills enhancement (A/M Session 13) and needs clarification (A/M Session 14).

This model recognizes that relapse is possible (even likely) when moving through the stages of change. People often "recycle" through the stages many different times before reaching success; thus, a "slip" should not be considered an utter failure, but rather a step back. Many people progress from contemplation to action to maintenance, but some will relapse. Following a relapse, individuals often regress to an earlier stage and then begin progressing through the stages yet again. Frequently, people who do relapse have a better chance of success during the next cycle. They have often learned new ways to deal with old behaviors, and they now have a history of successes on which to build. It is important to help clients see a lapse as a temporary *slip* rather than a failure, and to realize that many people cycle though the stages a number of times before they are able to maintain successful behavior change.

HOW THE PROCESSES FACILITATE
MOVEMENT THROUGH THE STAGES

As Prochaska, Norcross, and DiClemente explain in *Changing for Good* (1994), "Any activity that you initiate to help modify your thinking, feeling, or behavior is a change process" (p. 25). While not all of the processes are used by all therapies, each type of intervention produces change by applying certain processes. Likewise, when people change on their own, they use these processes.

The early stage processes, particularly *consciousness-raising* and *self-reevaluation*, involve raising awareness of the problem behavior. This awareness is critical in that once a person has insight into a behavior, he or she is more likely to make intelligent decisions about changing. Most of the major therapies begin by trying to raise a person's level of awareness about the problem behavior, but many interventions stop at that point. Research on the use of the processes of change shows that once a person has become aware of the problem, it is important that he or she consider the pros and cons of the behavior. An assessment of the "good things" and the "not so good things" about substance use, for example, helps clients to get a clearer picture of their reasons for use as well as what it might be like if they change the behavior. Using the change process of *self-reevaluation*, the client also begins to assess how the problem affects his or her life and, through *social liberation*, sees how society supports alternative, healthier behaviors. This is the point at which clients see how the problem behavior conflicts with personal values and begin to think about how life might be different once they have altered the behavior. By using *environmental reevaluation*, they also begin to become aware of how their behavior affects those around them. Thus, each of the early stage processes are related to one another, and, collectively, they are important in facilitating movement through the stages of change.

It should be noted that while the change process of *social liberation* has typically been viewed as being most salient in the early stages of change, it is also important in the later stages. In the contemplation stage, social liberation comes into play when the individual begins to notice ways in which society provides alternatives to the problem behavior (e.g., providing nonsmoking areas, promoting designated drivers). In the action and maintenance stages, people often strive to alter their social environment in ways that can help them maintain the changes they have made (e.g., joining a 12-step group, participating in job training programs). In the later stages, social liberation lends support to personally empowering behaviors and increases clients' self-esteem as they come to believe in their own power to change.

While the early stage processes are relatively distinct, three of the later stage processes, namely, stimulus control, counterconditioning, and reinforcement management, often function together. For the purposes of this intervention, it is useful to understand how these three processes are linked.

The change processes of stimulus control, counterconditioning, and reinforcement management are based on two fundamental psychological theories of learning that view behavior as being controlled in large measure by the environment. You will remember these theories by Pavlov and Skinner from your early psychology courses. The first theory, generated by Ivan Pavlov, describes how antecedent cues in the environment can become powerful triggers for behavior. Pavlov discovered that many behaviors involve "conditioning." A once-neutral cue (e.g., a bell) can become an automatic trigger for certain reactions (e.g., salivating). He demonstrated this principle by conditioning a dog to salivate when hearing a bell. He did this by first pairing the bell with food, and then removing the food. This same kind of conditioning can happen in humans. Drug and alcohol abusers give many examples of experiences, people, and places that have become closely linked to using and craving, and that subsequently serve as triggers to use.

The processes of stimulus control and counterconditioning are based on Pavlov's theory. The first, stimulus control, attempts to change the cues in the environment. Avoiding the people, places, and activities that trigger drug or alcohol use is a good example of this process. The second, counterconditioning, works to change the reaction to a stimulus. For example, anxiety and frustration are often cues to use alcohol or other drugs. A healthier response to the same feelings would be to do relaxation exercises. This represents the change process of counterconditioning.

The psychological theory developed by B. F. Skinner (1982) describes how conse-quences can affect behavior. Skinner detailed the idea that reinforced behaviors tend to occur more frequently. In terms of substance use, pleasurable reactions upon using a drug, as well as negative reactions when not using, can both act as reinforcers for con-tinuing to use. The change process that directly focuses on the consequence of behav-ior is reinforcement management. This process tries to change the reinforcers that can influence drug use or recovery. Having substance abusers congratulate themselves on their efforts not to use substances is a case of self-reinforcement. AA "sobriety chips" and birthdays, as well as finding alternative reinforcers that support sobriety, are exam-ples of other people or activities that are reinforcers in the environment. Also, the posi-tive results of making a behavior change can be reinforcing in and of themselves. For example, experiencing a positive result due to being assertive increases the likelihood that you will be assertive in the future because those skills have been reinforced by a success.

On a basic level, in order to change substance use behavior, the stimuli that pre-cede the behavior and the reinforcers that follow it must be changed. Figure 1.1 illus-trates how these processes function. Sometimes people can change or alter the stimulus that tempts them to use (e.g., avoid bars, remove drugs from the home). Some stimuli, however, may be difficult to avoid or alter (such as things that other people might say or do). In this case, it can be effective for clients to change *their responses* to the stimulus (i.e., use the change process of counterconditioning) rather than attempting to control it. In this way, clients can use counterconditioning either to change their internal re-sponses to cues (such as thoughts or emotions) or to substitute different behaviors when those cues prompt the internal response.

Notice that the change process of reinforcement management is also connected in Figure 1.1, with behavior and future behavior. As mentioned earlier, the positive conse-quences of a new behavior can be reinforcing in and of themselves, and can lead to maintenance of the behavior in the future. Clients can also receive "rewards" following a behavior change, such as tokens from AA or a note of encouragement from a friend. These reinforcers also increase the likelihood that the behavior will be repeated in the future.

Although these three processes—stimulus control, counterconditioning, and rein-

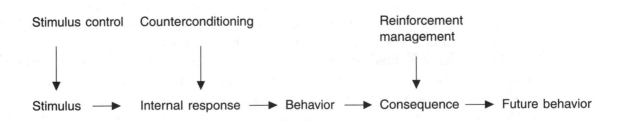

FIGURE 1.1. Three behavioral processes at work.

forcement management—are defined separately and there are intervention techniques that represent each one, often, interventions engage two or more processes at the same time. Going to an AA meeting, for example, can provide some stimulus control in keeping away from "drinking buddies" and also reinforcement management by the support and encouragement of a sponsor or fellow AA member. Thus, some of the later stage sessions in this manual give examples of activities that are both specific to one process and engage multiple processes at the same time.

The final two behavioral processes, *self-liberation* and *helping relationships*, involve making a commitment to change and utilizing the support necessary to make that change. This commitment and the "shoring up" of one's support network are crucial to navigating through the later stages on to successful maintenance.

THE DIFFERENCE BETWEEN PROCESSES OF CHANGE AND TECHNIQUES

There is an important distinction between the processes of change and techniques that can stimulate those processes. *For each process, there are dozens, even hundreds, of techniques.* What we have attempted to do in this manual is alert you to the processes most relevant to each stage of change and suggest specific techniques that will encourage clients' use of those processes. As Prochaska, Norcross, and DiClemente (1994) suggest, the matching of stage and process is a key to change. Once we know what stage an individual is in, we can assist that person in applying the processes that are necessary to move to the next stage through the use of various techniques.

ADAPTING THIS MANUAL TO YOUR NEEDS

The TTM's change processes drive this intervention and provide direction and structure, but their sequence and related techniques are not "cast in stone." The sophisticated clinician will be able to select those sessions that are most appropriate for a group or an individual at any particular stage or time in treatment. Once you are familiar with all of the processes of change, you will be able to recognize other techniques, beyond those included in this manual, that correspond to process movement. This manual provides the facilitator, with examples of specific techniques and exercises that correspond to each particular process, and some that cover multiple processes. Other materials (you are probably already familiar with many of them) offer techniques that can also be used to increase process use. The Appendix includes a list of other materials that we have found helpful in this regard.

CHAPTER 2

Strategies for Facilitating Change

Each of the 29 sessions in this manual has at least one particular change process as its focus, and the activities for that session are intended to strengthen that change process. Clinicians are guided through each session and told how to use the various session techniques to encourage use of the target process. At this point, however, we would like to emphasize that this is not a "cookbook" approach, but that it should be guided by an overarching counseling style that will increase clients' motivation for change.

A MOTIVATIONAL APPROACH

Motivation plays an important role in people's decision to change their substance use. In this model, motivation is viewed as something that can be influenced rather than a specific personality characteristic or trait. In fact, increasing client motivation is seen as a central part of the clinician's task. As mentioned previously, Miller and Rollnick (1991) have developed a style of intervention called "motivational interviewing" (MI), which complements the stages of change model. The data supporting the effectiveness of MI in various settings is growing (Miller, Benefield, & Tongian, 1993; Noonan & Moyers, 1997; Project MATCH Research Group, 1997).

While this manual does not use MI per se, *its effectiveness is greatly enhanced when the session content is delivered in an MI style.* For that reason, clinicians using this manual are encouraged to attend a training workshop in MI. (Contact information is provided in the Appendix.) Miller and Rollnick's book *Motivational Interviewing: Preparing People to Change Addictive Behavior* (1991) is also highly recommended (at the time of this writing, a second edition is in preparation). An additional excellent resource is a manual published by the Mid-Atlantic Addiction Technology Transfer Center entitled *Motivational Groups for Community Substance Abuse Programs* (Ingersoll, Wagner, & Gharib, 2000). A brief summary of MI is included in this chapter to provide some background in this counseling style and to demonstrate how it can be used to enhance clients' use of the processes of change.

The MI approach begins with the assumption that the responsibility and capability for change lies within the client. The counselor's task is to create a set of conditions that will enhance the client's motivation for and commitment to change.

PRINCIPLES OF MOTIVATIONAL INTERVIEWING

Miller and Rollnick have described five specific principles and five strategies that are key to the MI approach.

Express Empathy

In MI, the counselor actively listens to the client without judgment, criticism, or blame in order to gain a better understanding of his or her situation and perspective. The counselor understands that the client may not be ready or willing to give up substance use in the early stages. Thus, the initial focus is on building therapeutic rapport and supporting the client instead of verbally suggesting change.

Develop Discrepancy

One of the goals of MI is to create and amplify discrepancy in the client's mind between present and past behavior, and future goals. This is done through examination of the consequences of continued substance use (often, by looking at the pros of changing and the cons of remaining the same). The hope is that the client will then be able to present the argument for change and begin to realize the need for change.

Avoid Argumentation

MI differs from other approaches to treating substance use in that it does not label clients as "alcoholics" or "drug addicts." When the counselor senses resistance, it is time to change strategies. This is an important principle behind the success of instilling motivation. Most people will not be motivated to change if they feel they are not supported in their efforts and must defend their actions.

Roll with Resistance

When faced with resistance, it becomes important to let the resistance be expressed instead of trying to fight against it. It is helpful for the counselor to reflect the client's questions and concerns, so that the client may further examine the possible alternatives. Thus, the client becomes the source of the possible answers, does not feel defeated in sharing his or her concerns, and is able to take the risk to express feelings.

Support Self-Efficacy

The counselor can support the client's confidence in his or her ability to change in a variety of ways. One of these ways is to present the client with examples of positive changes he or she has made, while another is to emphasize the importance of taking responsibility. Finally, clients should feel strong support and a positive rapport with the facilitator, which furthers their sense of self-efficacy.

USING MOTIVATIONAL INTERVIEWING TO ENHANCE CHANGE PROCESS USE

As the stages of change illustrate, many clients are not yet ready or motivated to change. If they were, it would be appropriate to introduce skills development and other action-related tasks immediately. Too often, past treatment approaches have tried to help people change by simply "teaching" or lecturing. While clinicians had a rich repertoire of techniques to use for clients in the more action-oriented stages, they were at a loss as to what to do with precontemplators or contemplators.

It is clear, however, that if clients are not yet ready to change their problem behaviors (i.e., precontemplators), then clinicians need to use an approach that raises their awareness of the need to change in a nonthreatening way. Therefore, the goal of MI is to *prepare people for change*, not necessarily to push them into changing. The motivational approach encourages use of the early stage processes of change by helping people work through their ambivalence about changing. This is accomplished through the use of active listening and gentle feedback techniques.

While each session in this manual offers specific techniques to enhance process use, these techniques are optimized when they are applied using a motivational style. For example, simply giving information does not necessarily result in consciousness raising. A client is much more likely to hear and absorb the information when it is delivered in a way that is respectful, nonconfrontational, empathetic, and based on that particular client's needs. In this way, clients are guided through the early stages and learn to use the various related processes in a manner that is tailored to their specific readiness to change.

It is also important to note that MI is useful in promoting process use in the later stages. While the focus is somewhat different, and the clinician no longer has to concentrate on building motivation for change, the counseling style is still important in that it helps to increase clients' self-efficacy and to firm their commitment to change. For instance, in counterconditioning, rather than the counselor suggesting alternatives to substance use, clients are encouraged to generate alternatives that are specific to their situation and needs. In this way, the client builds a plan that is individualized, and one that he or she is more likely to follow over the long term.

Unlike traditional approaches to treatment, which often provoke resistance, the goal of the motivational approach is to reduce resistance and motivate the client for change. In this approach, the counselor works to elicit the client's own concerns. When the client (rather than the counselor) articulates the reasons for change, the client's internal motivation is harnessed and he or she is more ready to change. The majority of work in MI involves exploring clients' ambivalence, or mixed feelings, about change, and matching interventions to their current level of readiness for change.

In summary, MI is a very effective counseling style for working with clients in the early stages of change, because it facilitates client motivation. However, it is also an important style to use in the later stage sessions. Although the later stage sessions are more action-oriented, clients still do better when approached with an empathetic, caring style. For these clients, MI helps increase self-efficacy and reinforces their accomplishments, both of which are important to the action and maintenance stages of change.

We highlight Miller and Rollnick's principles and next, the specific MI strategies, because they fit beautifully within the framework of the TTM. We have tried to build these elements into the group sessions as much as possible. One example of this is the provision of feedback. Although providing individualized feedback to each client is not feasible within the group context, we have clients in the early stages (P/C/P Sessions 3 and 4) self-administer and score the Alcohol Use Disorders Identification Test and the Drug Screening Inventory. The same technique is used in a later session, with temptation and confidence items from the Alcohol Abstinence Self-Efficacy Scale (DiClemente, Carbonari, & Hughes, 1994) (AASE-A; P/C/P Session 11). The group facilitator discusses the meaning of each range of scores, enabling clients to receive information about their own situation while maintaining their privacy.

You will notice that the emphasis shifts from a more motivational approach in the early stage sessions (P/C/P Sessions 1–14) to one that is behavioral or "action-oriented" in the later stage sessions (A/M Sessions 1–15). It is important to note that you do not abandon use of motivational techniques as clients move into the later stages, but rather incorporate the motivational style into a somewhat more traditional cognitive-behavioral or relapse-prevention approach.

MOTIVATIONAL STRATEGIES

A motivational approach is one that is nonconfrontational and includes components of empathy, respect, and a belief in the power of self-motivation. The following strategies specified by Miller and Rollnick (1991) will be helpful in maintaining an empathetic and motivational style in each session of this intervention:

1. *Ask open-ended questions.* Ask questions that cannot easily be answered with a "yes" or "no." With ambivalent clients, ask for both positive and negative aspects of the problem.

2. *Listen reflectively.* Reflective listening involves forming a reasonable guess as to the meaning of clients' statements and giving voice to this guess in the form of a statement. Realize that what you believe or assume people to mean is not necessarily what they really mean, and reflect words as well as emotions.

3. *Affirm.* Affirm and support the client's efforts to change with compliments and

statements of appreciation and understanding. This reinforcement will increase self-efficacy and increase the likelihood that the client will continue to move toward change.

4. *Summarize.* Periodic summaries link together discussed material, demonstrate careful listening, prepare clients to move on, and are especially good for examining ambivalence around an issue. At the end of a session, it is useful to offer a major summary, clearly and succinctly pulling together what has transpired.

Many of the techniques used in these sessions will be familiar to you; most of them are not unique in substance abuse treatment. However, the value of this intervention lies in applying techniques specific to a particular process in a manner that is tailored to the client's stage of change, and in delivering this intervention in a motivational manner.

OVERVIEW OF TECHNIQUES

The sessions in this manual utilize a number of traditional psychotherapeutic techniques in order to assist clients in progressing through the stages of change. These techniques are based on different systems of psychological theory and have been applied in numerous settings. What is unique about this manual, however, is the coupling of established tools and strategies with particular processes of change. The likelihood that clients will engage in process use is increased by conducting group activities using techniques that enhance use of relevant processes at specific points during treatment.

Table 2.1 details the various techniques that are utilized throughout the manual as they relate to the processes of change and their respective session topics. What follows is a brief description of each technique, as well as examples of empirical support for technique efficacy.

Psychoeducation

Although clinicians frequently provide information to their clients in a variety of ways, psychoeducation (a didactic style of teaching psychologically relevant information) is one of the most beneficial. Psychoeducation has been found to be an effective tool in a number of settings (Kominars, 1997; Malow, West, Corrigan, Pena, & Cunningham, 1994). In this manual, this technique enhances the change processes of consciousness raising, stimulus control, and social liberation by providing information regarding substance use and its potential effects in a motivational style.

Values Clarification

The goal of this technique is to have clients define their values system, as well as to identify the things that they value most in life. In doing so, many clients realize that their substance use is discrepant with their values and begin to consider making changes in their substance use. This has been found to be an effective tool in a substance-using population (Friedman & Utada, 1992). In this intervention, the technique

TABLE 2.1. Techniques Used to Enhance Process Movement

Process of change	Session topic(s)	Technique(s)
Consciousness raising	Daily usage Physiological effects Expressions of concern	Assessment/feedback Psychoeducation Cognitive recognition
Self-reevaluation	Expectations of use Values	Cognitive recognition Values clarification
Decisional balance[a]	Weighing pros and cons	Decision making
Environmental reevaluation	Relationships Roles	Cognitive recognition Role clarification
Efficacy[a]	Confidence and temptation Problem solving	Problem solving
Self-liberation	Goals Action plan Recommitting after a slip	Goal setting Relapse prevention planning Framing
Stimulus control	Triggers	Psychoeducation Environmental restructuring
Counterconditioning	Stress Assertiveness Refusal skills Thought management	Relaxation imagery Assertion Role play Cognitive restructuring
Reinforcement management	Rewarding success Cravings and urges Alternatives to using	Reinforcement Cognitive restructuring
Helping relationships	Social support	Social skills enhancement Communication skills
Social liberation	Identifying needs and resources	Needs clarification Psychoeducation

[a]While decisional balance and self-efficacy are not considered to be processes of change, they are key process components in the stages of change model.

of values clarification is used to enhance the change process of self reevaluation. Specifically, clients in this intervention are asked to define their values and then examine how their substance use is discrepant with those values.

Problem Solving

Many clients who abuse alcohol and other drugs have poor problem-solving skills. By enhancing clients' ability to logically and rationally think through a situation, generate potential alternatives (i.e., brainstorm), and then select the most appropriate solution, clinicians provide crucial life skills that help clients solve substance-related as well as everyday problems. General problem-solving guidelines used in education, business, and counseling settings can be found in numerous sources. Montl, Abrams, Kadden, and Cooney (1989) provide guidelines specific to substance abusing clients. The technique of problem solving is used in this intervention to enhance self-efficacy.

Goal Setting

As is the case with problem solving, many clients are unable to establish goals effectively and then follow through on the steps by which to attain these goals. This technique is designed to teach clients the difference between a realistic goal and one that is unattainable, and to facilitate their creation of substance-related goals. Miller (1985, 1987, 1989) has repeatedly stressed the importance of increasing appropriate goal setting in substance-abusing populations, as have numerous other clinicians (Hester, 1995; McMurran, 1996; Wing, 1991). Goal setting is used in this intervention to enhance the change process of self-liberation by encouraging clients to develop and commit to substance-related goals.

Relapse Prevention Planning

In working with clients who abuse alcohol and other drugs, it is important to have them proactively plan for times when they are tempted to use by writing down the exact actions they can take when tempted. Research has shown that such plans can be highly effective in preventing further substance use. For an extensive discussion of relapse prevention theory, research, and practice, refer to Marlatt and Gordon's (1985) book *Relapse Prevention*. In this manual, relapse prevention planning is used to assist clients in developing an "action" plan, thus enhancing the change process of self-liberation by encouraging clients to make a commitment to change.

Relaxation Techniques

Often, clients use substances to relieve anxiety or other negative emotions. Relaxation techniques arc useful in helping clients calm themselves down when they are faced with stressful situations that might trigger substance use. The goal is to teach clients how to systematically relax their bodies and their minds using stress-reduction and imagery techniques. There are a number of books available on stress reduction and relaxation (e.g., Benson, 1975; Kabat-Zinn, 1990). Relaxation techniques taught in this manual allow for replacement of anxiety with calmness and awareness, thus enhancing the change process of counterconditioning.

Assertion Training

One of the most tempting situations for clients who struggle with alcohol and other drug abuse is when they are offered a substance by another person. Assertion training provides the clients with the skills they need in order to successfully turn down an offer to use. This technique involves teaching clients how to use positive body language and assertive statements in order to convey their meaning to others. Botvin and Wills (1985) reported that training in social assertiveness skills results in significant effects on substance abuse behaviors. The assertiveness training in this manual enhances the change process of counterconditioning by providing healthy responses for clients to substitute in place of substance use in tempting situations.

Role Play

By having clients "act out" situations before they occur, facilitators are helping group members to anticipate how they might feel, act, and react in those same situations. Role plays can be extremely powerful and beneficial in assisting clients with practicing new ways of speaking and acting. Rohrbach, Graham, Hansen, and Flay (1987) reported that subjects who engage in role plays during treatment perform better on a skills measure and show greater alcohol refusal self-efficacy than do subjects who do not participate in role plays. Role plays assist in the practice new behaviors that enhance the change process of counterconditioning by providing alternate behaviors to substitute in place of substance use in tempting situations.

Cognitive Techniques

For many substance-abusing clients, it is important to change thinking patterns regarding alcohol and other drugs. Several cognitive techniques are used throughout this intervention, including cognitive restructuring, recognition, and framing. Cognitive restructuring involves teaching clients to recognize thoughts that could lead to substance use, then explaining how to replace those thoughts with healthier drug- and alcohol-avoidant ones. Recognition involves teaching clients to recognize relationships, situations, and perspectives that they may have previously overlooked or ignored. Finally, the technique of framing involves teaching clients how to view situations in a healthier, more realistic manner. Extensive empirical support exists for the efficacy of cognitive techniques, especially with regard to substance-abusing clients (Kadden et al., 1995; Carroll, 1998). Cognitive techniques are important to both the experiential and the behavioral processes of change. By providing tools for clients to change their maladaptive cognitions and incorrect perspectives, several change processes are enhanced, including consciousness raising, self reevaluation, environmental reevaluation, self-liberation, counterconditioning, and reinforcement management.

Environmental Restructuring

The goal of this technique is to encourage clients to alter or avoid situations in which they are tempted to use alcohol or other drugs. By making significant changes in the situations in which they function daily, the likelihood that clients will avoid further substance use is increased. This technique enhances the change process of stimulus control by assisting clients with altering or avoiding tempting situations, thereby limiting exposure to triggers.

Role Clarification

Although this technique is frequently used in organizational psychology to diffuse conflict between coworkers or other systems relationships, it can be beneficial when working with substance abusers as well. The goal is to have clients identify the numerous roles that they play (e.g., father, son, coworker, church member), and then determine how their substance use has affected those roles. This technique enhances the change process of environmental reevaluation by assisting clients in recognizing how their substance use has affected the environments in which they function.

Reinforcement

Perhaps one of the most empirically studied techniques is reinforcement. The theory, developed by B. F. Skinner, is that when a behavior is rewarded, the likelihood that it will occur again is increased. Numerous clinicians have endorsed the use of reinforcement when working with substance abusing clients (e.g., Higgins, 1999; Higgins & Silverman, 1999; Bigelow, Brooner, & Silverman, 1998). This technique exemplifies the change process of reinforcement management.

Social Skills and Communication Skills Enhancement

As is the case with several daily life skills, substance-abusing clients often have difficulties with both social and communication skills. Teaching clients how to communicate effectively with others, while simultaneously respecting others' space, perspectives, and beliefs, will benefit clients greatly. Monti and O'Leary (1999) advocate for the implementation of coping and social skills training in interventions working with alcohol and cocaine-dependent clients. Monti et al.'s book *Treating Alcohol Dependence* (1989) discusses theory and research on coping skills, along with many other social skills exercises. In this manual, social and communication skills training enhance the change process of helping relationships by providing clients with skills that result in the expansion of their support system.

Needs Clarification

Due to the overwhelming repercussions of substance abuse, many clients neglect taking care of important areas of their lives. A needs clarification exercise is designed to assist clients in reviewing various areas of their lives and identifying those in which they could use improvement. This technique enhances the change process of social liberation by assisting clients with identifying resources that can be utilized to maintain changes and improve various areas of their lives.

Assessment and Feedback

Although assessment is not, by definition, a therapeutic technique, assessment and the provision of feedback often provides clients with the opportunity to look realistically at the extent of their substance use. One excellent assessment instrument is the Timeline Followback (TLFB). Developed by Linda and Mark Sobell (1992), the goal of the TLFB is to help clients gain a realistic picture of the extent of their substance use. In administering the assessment, the clinician asks clients to describe their drinking or drug use during a certain time period. By detailing their substance use during different parts of a day, month, or year, clients often learn that they are using more than they had originally realized. They may also be able to identify the times when they are most likely to use (e.g., during "happy hour" at the local bar, or during certain holiday periods). This technique enhances the change process of consciousness raising by helping clients realize the extent that they are using substances.

In summary, this manual utilizes a number of empirically based, conventional therapeutic techniques in order to help clients understand and engage in the processes of change and, by doing so, subsequently progress through the stages of change.

CHAPTER 3

Putting It All Together: Setting Up and Carrying Out the Intervention

OVERVIEW OF THIS TREATMENT

As mentioned in the Introduction, the sessions in this manual are organized into two separate group sequences, with 14 and 15 sessions, respectively. The first sequence (P/C/P Sessions 1–14) is designed for those in the early stages of change (precontemplation, contemplation, and preparation). The second sequence (A/M Sessions 1–15) is designed for those in the later stages of change (action and maintenance). We chose a group format for this manual because most treatment facilities prefer to use a group modality for treatment delivery. Our goal was to respond to the needs of the treatment community and to make this manual as adaptable to the needs of various agencies as possible. For those clinicians who have the luxury of providing more individual and tailored treatment, each session can be easily adapted. Sessions can also "stand alone," enabling the clinician to tailor the work to the needs of the group and/or the individual. It is possible to alter the sequence or overall number of sessions as appropriate to your clients and setting. For instance, if the majority of your group seems familiar with relaxation techniques, you might simply highlight the main points of those particular sessions and continue on to the next topic. For some sessions, you may need to incorporate some of the main points from the sessions you "skip" into those that the group does complete.

At intake, clients are assessed for their stage status and assigned to the group appropriate for their stage. In some cases, the change desired may be reduction of substance use; in most other cases, it is abstinence.

Clients can be moved from one group to the other depending on their progression or regression through the stages of change. For those clients who are not progressing through the stages, some repetition of sessions or, ultimately, a more individualized form of treatment may be required. After the intake sessions and assignment to group, therapists should continue to evaluate the client's progress and make decisions about whether and when a client moves from one group to the other.

For those settings where there is enough of a client flow to fill multiple groups, the best strategy is to have two groups (one in each sequence) running simultaneously. One group covers the early stages of change (P/C/P), while the other covers the later stages (A/M). These groups may be open, accepting new members when they arrive, and continuously repeated. Clients in the first group could be moved up as soon as judged ready.

An alternative system is to assign clients to groups based on stage at intake and to keep them in that group through the entire session sequence. This strategy is preferable where closed groups are desired. We prefer that groups be closed (i.e., no new members admitted once the group has begun), but this manual can be used in either open or closed groups.

WHO SHOULD CONDUCT THIS TREATMENT?

Although this intervention is not designed to delve deeply into psychological issues and problems, it does require training and skill. Optimally, it is suggested that the facilitator be a licensed counselor, psychologist, or social worker (master's degree or higher), a licensed chemical dependency counselor, or have a number of years facilitating groups under the supervision of the above. If this approach is used in a group format, it is important that the facilitator be someone who has been trained in leading groups.

It would also be helpful to be well versed in the TTM when using this manual in groups or individually. A recent book entitled *Treating Alcohol and Drug Problems: Working within the Stages of Change Model* (Connors, Donovan, & DiClemente, 2001) is an excellent resource and provides detailed descriptions of the various components of the model, as well as guidelines for using the model for treatment planning, individual and group treatment, and with special populations. There are also numerous research articles available on the model. The References section at the back of this manual can direct you to some of these. *Changing for Good* (Prochaska, Norcross, & DiClemente, 1994) can provide you with additional information about how the stages and processes work together. Attendance at a workshop or seminar on the TTM is also encouraged (contact information is provided in the Appendix). As mentioned earlier, training in MI is also available. In addition, the book *Motivational Interviewing: Preparing People to Change Addictive Behavior*, by Miller and Rollnick (1991), is highly recommended reading for facilitators; *however, it does not take the place of attending the training workshops.* Contact information for these trainings is also in the Appendix.

IN WHAT SETTINGS IS THIS TREATMENT APPROPRIATE?

This intervention is designed to be useful in a variety of settings and, because of its flexibility, can prove effective with a wide range of clients. Examples of potential settings are inpatient treatment programs and/or residential treatment facilities, outpatient treatment programs, social service agencies, mental health agencies, youth facilities, college campuses, assisted-living centers, ex-offender programs, and criminal justice settings.

SUGGESTED GROUP SIZE, FREQUENCY OF SESSIONS, AND SESSION LENGTH

Most of the literature on facilitating groups recommends an optimal group size of 8–12 members. Our experience is consistent with this. As the goal is to assist clients in moving through the stages, it is important that groups meet regularly and frequently in order to keep these new thoughts, behaviors, and emotions alive. We suggest twice-weekly groups but urge facilitators to observe what works best for their particular group—three times a week may be best in particular settings, while in other settings, more than once a week may put a burden on members. If time is an issue, you may want to select those sessions that you judge would be most beneficial to your clients. Sessions are designed to be conducted within a 1-hour time period. However, with larger groups, 90-minute sessions may prove more workable.

INTAKE SCREENING AND ASSESSMENT

There are several methods for assessing clients' stage of change and a number of issues involved in assigning clients to groups based on stage. We first briefly review three possible methods of assessing stage of change: the Readiness Ruler, the clinical interview, and the University of Rhode Island Change Assessment Scale (URICA) questionnaire. While we offer guidance in this area, again, we encourage you to find the method that works best for you.

Methods of Assessment

1. The *Readiness Ruler* (shown in Figure 3.1) offers a quick and simple way of assessing stage. The clinician shows the client the ruler and simply asks, "Which point on this line best reflects how ready you are at the present time to change your drinking/drug use?" Be sure the term "change" is defined so that it is clear to the client the type of change you are assessing (i.e., abstinence or reduction). This instrument is certainly the easiest to use. However, clients must believe that they can endorse any point on this ruler without being judged and that the purpose of this exercise is to assist in developing the best treatment plan for them. (If this tool is to be used, it is important that the philosophy of the program not be punitive and that clients understand that they will not be penalized if they endorse an earlier point on the ruler.)

Figure 3.1 is an example of a ruler used to assess a client's readiness to quit drinking. Each ruler should clearly specify the target behavior. For example, a client may be at one point for quitting drinking and yet another for quitting cocaine use, so readiness

Make a slash mark on the line that most closely expresses your answer to this question:
How ready are you *at the present time* to change your drinking?

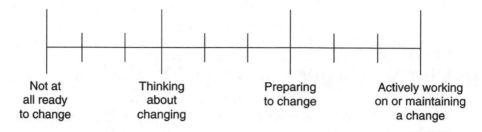

FIGURE 3.1. Readiness Ruler. From Velasquez, Maurer, Crouch, and DiClemente (2001). Copyright by The Guilford Press. Permission to photocopy this handout is granted to purchasers of this book for professional use only (see copyright page for details).

rulers should be completed for both behaviors. Likewise, if the target behavior is for an outcome other than abstinence, such as a reduction in drinking, the client should be clear about the target outcome. For example, in one study we are conducting, the target behavior is for clients to drink below "risky levels" as defined by the National Institute on Alcohol Abuse and Alcoholism. In that case, we define risky levels (for women, no more than 4 drinks on one occasion or no more than 7 drinks in one week). In other cases, the client sets the drinking goal prior to completing the readiness ruler. This instrument is designed to be adaptable to many behaviors, and the key to using it effectively is to be very clear about the target behavior.

2. A *clinical interview* is another way to assess a client's stage of change. The challenge for this type of assessment is one of gaining an accurate understanding of client stage status. How can the therapist accurately assess stage? By asking the client to talk about substance use and any associated problems, the clinician can determine where a client is in terms of motivation to change. For example, a client in the precontemplation stage might say, "My drinking does not cause problems. I am only here because my probation officer says I have to be in a program." Clients in precontemplation may become defensive when asked about their substance use. Clients in the contemplation stage are considering the pros and cons of change. They might be wondering what their lives might be like if they change their substance use. They often want more information about the problem and what it might take to change. Clients in the preparation stage may indicate that they are planning to make changes in their substance use, while clients in the action stage have already made some changes (such as a brief quit attempt or avoiding places where they would be exposed to drugs or alcohol). Clients in the maintenance stage have already quit their problem behavior and are trying to maintain the change.

A sensitive discussion of the client's readiness to change is the easiest and most efficient way to track stage for a particular client. However, as any clinician will tell you, judgments about any particular client at any specific time can be erroneous. Settings where clients feel that they must give right answers or tell you what you want to hear interfere with their making and sharing accurate self-appraisals. Clinical judgments based on quick impressions, biased assumptions, and poor listening often are responsible for inaccurate evaluation of the client. To accurately assess stage of change, the therapist must allow the client to be open and listen to what he or she is thinking and doing with respect to the problem. This information can be used independently of other measures, or concurrently to validate the data collected using the URICA (discussed next) or the Readiness Ruler.

3. The *University of Rhode Island Change Assessment Scale* (URICA; McConnaughy, DiClemente, Prochaska, & Velicer, 1989) is a self-administered questionnaire consisting of a series of items that can vary from 12 to 32, depending on which form of the instrument is being used. The items represent four stage-of-change subscales: precontemplation (PC), contemplation (C), action (A), and maintenance (M). A preparation scale was developed but failed to emerge as an independent factor, so is not used in the URICA. The URICA has a 5-point Likert-type-scale format through which participants rate the degree to which they agree or disagree with each of the items. Once mean scores are calculated on each subscale, they can be used as indicators of stage status in a number of ways. One approach is to create clusters of individuals with different profiles across the subscales (DiClemente & Hughes, 1991). The subscales can also be summed (C + A + M minus PC) to form a readiness score that can be compared to various ranges of scores (DiClemente & Prochaska, 1998).

The URICA is the best instrument to use for research and evaluation with substance abusing clients. Since it requires scoring and comparison with norms, it is best to use the URICA in settings where there is statistical expertise. When assessing stage for clinical purposes, we recommend that you use the Readiness Ruler in item 1.

Special Considerations

Assessing stage status can also be complicated by the reality that an individual client may be in different stages for different types of substances. We know, for example, that many methadone maintenance clients are actively working to stop using heroin but can be in very early stages for stopping other types of drug use, such as marijuana or cocaine. Or clients may be convinced that they need to quit using cocaine but believe that they have no serious drinking problem. In this case, they would be in the preparation or action stage for cocaine but in the precontemplation stage for changing their drinking. Clinicians need to not only evaluate the stage of change for the primary substance abuse problem but also examine the stage for other drugs of abuse and other problems. Our suggestion is that therapists focus primarily on the stage of change for the client's primary substance abuse problem in the group therapy, keeping in mind that each client may be in a different stage for other problems.

Assigning Clients to Groups

Once the therapist has evaluated stage status of each of the potential group members, the challenge becomes how to create the most effective group and assign clients to the group. In general, when organizing therapy groups, a therapist can create more homogeneous or heterogeneous groups with respect to stage status of participants, type of substance abused, and other considerations (gender, age). The group sessions outlined in this manual are for clients who are similar in their stage of change. Exercises are geared to assist individuals in certain stages of change and use specific processes of change to move them forward through the stages. For that reason, it is recommended that the groups consist of individuals either from the early stages of precontemplation and contemplation or those in the later stages of action and maintenance. Depending on the clinician's judgment, preparation-stage clients can be placed in either group. In general, we recommend that individuals in the preparation stage be placed with the precontemplation–contemplation–preparation group. Preparers can benefit from reinforcing their reasons for change via the experiential processes in the P/C/P group. In the latter sessions of this sequence, clients develop change plans to help them prepare for successful change. However, some clients in preparation might benefit more from placement in the action–maintenance group so that other group members can model change efforts and assist them in development of their plans to change.

A particular consideration is the placement of precontemplation and contemplation clients. In most settings, those clients in the precontemplation stage will be there due to some sort of legal mandate or pressure from family members or employers. It is important to recognize that while these external "motivators" may be central to the client's enrollment in the program, they do not assure investment in the change process. However, if the early stage group is facilitated in an accepting and skillful way, resistance to change is often minimized and clients become more aware of their own reasons for change.

In addition, when explaining the program to potential clients who express reluctance to change, it is important to emphasize that the program is meant to help them think through their own situation and consider what, if anything, they might want to do about their substance use. Assure them that no one will try to make them change. While they may be offered information, and maybe some advice, what they do with all of that is completely up to them. You might also tell them that other members of their group will be similar in terms of their readiness to change. When approached in this manner, clients in contemplation, and even precontemplation, are likely to be more receptive to participation in the program.

SESSION FORMAT

For ease of use, each session in this manual is presented in a consistent format. In each session you will find the following headings and information in the following order:

• *Change process objective.* We begin each session by stating the primary objective for that session, which is always a change process. For example, the change process objective for P/C/P Session 1 is "consciousness-raising." These change processes, including decisional balance and self-efficacy, promote client movement toward either preparation (for clients the P/C/P sequence) or maintenance (for clients in the A/M sequence).

• *Rationale.* This section briefly states why the sessions objectives are important and explains how they will be accomplished. For example, the rationale for P/C/P Session 2 explains that clients in the early stages of change are often unaware of how much or how often they abuse substances; this session helps raise clients' consciousness by asking them to describe usage over a typical day.

- *Content objectives.* Under this heading is a brief description of the content focus for the session (i.e., what you want the client to accomplish in the session). For example, the specific content objective for P/C/P Session 2 is that clients gain an awareness of the quantity, frequency, and patterns of their own substance use.

- *Materials required.* Most sessions call for distribution of client handouts or exercise forms. All such forms are contained in this book, at the end of each respective session, and they may be photocopied for client distribution. You will need to make copies in advance of the session and bring them to the group. This section alerts you to what you may need to be prepared in advance of each session.

- *Session summary.* Under this heading, you will find a brief overview of the main activities for that session.

- *Implementation.* This section discusses in more detail how to implement the session tasks, including practical tips and other procedural advice. For example, under the implementation section for P/C/P Session 2, you will learn that if clients have trouble identifying a "typical day" of substance use you can ask them to focus on a recent day of use. Specific questions to help prompt group discussions are also given.

- *Step-by-step session tasks.* In this section, you will find an outline for how to conduct the session that itemizes your tasks into sequential steps. Sessions always open with a brief check-in with the group (Step 1). The main topic is then introduced (Step 2). Further steps may include distributing handouts, guiding an activity, and leading a group discussion of the activity. Sessions always close with a brief group check-in and summary of the session.

It is *strongly* recommended that you refer to the implementation section in each session the first few times you facilitate the group. Once you become familiar with the details of the intervention, you can then use the step-by-step session tasks as a checklist of things to do during the course of each session, consulting the implementation text as needed.

BRIEF REFRESHER ON GROUP WORK

This may be your 100th group to lead or it may be your first. In either case, it will be helpful to review some basic techniques and guides for leading groups. Effective group management is an extensive topic in and of itself. However, the following overview explains the most relevant therapist issues and concerns in group work.

Leading Groups

The approach in this manual promotes certain elements that make it a natural fit for group work. For example, the likelihood that group members will be functioning in different (but closely related) stages of change throughout the course of a group means that members can benefit from the experiences of others yet not feel coerced or pressured to change.

As a group facilitator, it is your responsibility to assist and nurture the group. Using a motivational approach, remember, it is *not* your responsibility to create change; this is up to the client. In facilitating the group, there are three functions that you as leader should keep in mind, namely, creating the group, shaping the group, and maintaining the group.

In *creating* the group, remember that (in most cases) you are the single common element among all the group members. This is why they initially look to you for leadership and interaction.

In *shaping* the group, your experience and behavior, as well as the expectations of group members, will guide the formation of norms (i.e., rules for behavior in the group). You can shape norms both directly (by leading discussions of appropriate and inappropriate behavior) and indirectly (using verbal and nonverbal reinforcement; redirecting questions to the group rather than responding yourself; modeling acceptance, honesty, and genuineness). Keep in mind that norms are established early in the course of a group and are not easily changed subsequently (Yalom, 1995). The ideal group has norms that allow the processes of change to operate with maximum effectiveness, while respecting all members' uniqueness. Examples of helpful norms are the following:

- Nonjudgmental acceptance of others
- Willingness to self-disclose
- Participation by all group members
- Respecting confidentiality
- Valuing the importance of the group
- Recognizing the available support in the group
- Respecting others (using constructive criticism, no "name-calling")
- Willingness to accept feedback

These group norms are all consistent with a motivational approach to treatment, and the formation of these norms will help shape the motivational "spirit" of the group.

In *maintaining* the group, you function as a caretaker of sorts, handling issues that might arise that threaten group cohesion. Examples include subgrouping (the forming of "cliques" within the group), scapegoating, tardiness, members who "drop out," a crisis during a session, or breaches in confidentiality.

Group Facilitation Techniques

Two helpful references for group facilitation techniques are Yalom (1995) and Bertcher (1993). Other relevant group therapy principles, adapted from Yalom (1995), include the following:

- *Maintain a safe environment.* As the facilitator, it is your responsibility to ensure that clients feel not only physically safe but also emotionally safe enough to make self-disclosures to the group. One way to do this is to emphasize the importance of confidentiality among the group members. Once clients believe that what is spoken during group sessions actually does remain only within the group, they will be more likely to be open and honest with their statements. Another way to maintain a safe environment is to discourage inappropriate remarks and interactions, making sure that group members understand the difference between personal attacks and constructive criticism. It will be important to help the group establish such norms during the initial session and to model appropriate interactions throughout the course of the group.

• *Serve as group historian.* It is frequently useful in a group setting to help clients make connections between the present and previous sessions. Often, clients may not realize that their recent statements or behaviors are similar to those of other group members from previous sessions, and the illumination of these commonalities can be quite powerful. In addition, emphasize the mutual helpfulness of group members to one another and point out that the responsibility for change lies among themselves—not on you as the facilitator.

• *Help clients remain in the "here and now."* Many clients who have abused alcohol and other drugs for extended amounts of time tend to dwell on their past rather than focusing on the present or the future. Group settings provide a unique opportunity through which clients can help one another stop reliving the past, while they pay attention to their current situations. As a facilitator, it is helpful to assist clients in pointing out the following four things to one another:

1. This is an example of what your current behavior is like.
2. This is how your behavior makes others feel.
3. This is how your behavior influences others around you.
4. How does your behavior influence your opinion of yourself?

Again, keep in mind that just as in individual treatment, the *client* is the change agent in a group intervention that uses a motivational approach. The group and the facilitator provide a safe, supportive environment in which clients can explore their potential for change and gain the skills and confidence necessary to execute change.

CONCLUSION

We think you and your clients will find the group sessions in this manual to be informative, motivational, and fun. Because they are based on the latest research and techniques in the addictions field and are quite different from traditional treatment approaches, they may feel unfamiliar at first. As you begin to use this intervention, you will notice a somewhat different response by your clients than you have seen in the past. Since you will be working with clients "where they are" in terms of readiness to change, it is likely that they will be less resistant and more willing to draw upon their own resources and intrinsic motivations to change. Good luck as you and your clients move through the stages of change.

PART II

Thinking about Changing Substance Use

P/C/P Sequence:
Precontemplation–Contemplation–Preparation

CLIENT HANDOUTS

P/C/P-1.1. Stages of Change, 45

P/C/P-1.2. Where Am I?, 46

P/C/P-2.1. A Day in the Life, 51

P/C/P-3.1. Alcohol Use Disorders Identification Test (AUDIT), 56

P/C/P-3.2. Scoring the AUDIT, 57

P/C/P-3.3. AUDIT—What Does It Mean?, 58

P/C/P-3.4. What Can Alcohol Do?, 59

P/C/P-4.1. Drug Screening Inventory, 66

P/C/P-4.2. Scoring the Drug Screening Inventory, 67

P/C/P-4.3. What Can Drugs Do?, 68

P/C/P-5.1. My Expectations about Substance Use, 74

P/C/P-6.1. Who Is Concerned?, 79

P/C/P-7.1. What I Value Most in Life, 83

P/C/P-8.1. Carolyn's Pros and Cons for Alcohol Use, 89

P/C/P-8.2. My Pros and Cons for Substance Use, 90

P/C/P-9.1. My Relationships, 95

P/C/P-9.2. My Relationships (Example), 96

P/C/P-10.1. What Hats Do I Wear?, 101

P/C/P-11.1. The Most Tempting Times for Me Are . . . , 106

P/C/P-11.2. The Hardest Times for Me Are . . . , 107

P/C/P-12.1. Problem-Solving Examples, 111

P/C/P-12.2. Choosing a Solution: "Dave's Options", 112

P/C/P-13.1. Goal Setting and Change Plan (Example), 117

P/C/P-13.2. My Goal Setting and Change Plan, 118

P/C/P-14.1. Review, 123

The Stages of Change

CHANGE PROCESS OBJECTIVE: CONSCIOUSNESS RAISING

RATIONALE

The stages of change offer an integrative framework for understanding and facilitating behavior change. The sessions in this sequence are for clients who may not be ready to think about changing their substance use, who have been contemplating making changes, and who are "getting ready" to change their substance use. It is important for clients to understand the stages of change model and where they are currently located in the change process. This is the first step for consciousness raising.

CONTENT OBJECTIVES

Clients learn Stages of Change model.
Clients complete staging exercise to determine their own stage of change.

MATERIALS REQUIRED

Chalkboard/flipchart
Chalk or markers
Copies of the following handouts for distribution to each group member:
    "Stages of Change" handout (P/C/P-1.1)
    "Where Am I?" handout (P/C/P-1.2)

SESSION SUMMARY

Explain to clients that you will be using a "motivational approach" in the group, which is quite different than any treatment experiences they may have had in the past. In introducing these motivational concepts to group members, you will be teaching them how to use this style in their interactions with one another. Since this is very different from other groups in which they may have participated, it might take a while for them to get used to the style of interaction, and they may need gentle reminders as you progress through the early sessions. During this session, the group rules are established, and the stages of change model is discussed. The facilitator reads vignettes for each of the stages aloud, having the clients choose which stage applies to each scenario. The clients complete a simple self-staging exercise.

IMPLEMENTATION

Many clients in the precontemplation or contemplation stages may be participating in the program as the result of pressure from others. It is important to recognize and acknowledge that they may be resistant to the idea of changing their substance use. There are several ways in which clients may demonstrate this resistance. They may be openly hostile, may refuse to engage in conversation about substance use, or may appear to be participating but be inwardly passive and resentful. The way to diffuse this resistance is to "roll" with it, using motivational strategies. One example would be to acknowledge that many of the group members may feel pressured to be there, and that these feelings are completely normal. Assure them that most members are probably feeling the same way, and that the group will give them a chance to explore their own feelings about their substance use with others in similar situations. (Miller & Rollnick, 1991, describe specific strategies for handling resistance using an MI approach.) Describing the stages of change and acknowledging that other group members are likely to be in the early stages can also help reduce client resistance.

Step 1: Open the Session and Introduce Motivational Approach

Begin this session by introducing yourself. Tell clients that you are here to help them learn more about themselves and decide whether there are any changes they would like to make. Assure them that while you have the knowledge and the skills to help them, ultimately, *if there is any changing to be done, they will be the ones to do it.* The responsibility for change is up to them, and you will not coerce them or try to force them to change in any way. Tell clients that you are the group "facilitator," but each client also plays an important role in helping other group members as you go through this process together. Explain that this is also the approach you would like for clients to take toward one another: "In this group, we will use the motivational approach. This means we will avoid confrontation and, rather, help facilitate change in one another through supportive interactions." The approach to be taken by all members of the group should be one of empathy, acceptance, and respect for individual differences. *Emphasize that, unlike some models of substance abuse treatment, this approach explicitly avoids confrontation.*

Ask each group member to introduce him- or herself and tell one thing he or she would like to get out of the group. Since this is likely to be a new approach to most clients, spend a few minutes discussing how this approach feels to them. You may wish to tell them that research shows that a supportive, empathetic approach to behavior change is much more effective than a confrontational one.

Step 2: Establish Group Rules

Introduce the need for basic group rules to help keep the group cohesive. The following rules have been found to be helpful in establishing a safe environment in which clients feel free to participate.

- Respect self and others in the group.
- Refrain from interrupting or talking when others are talking.
- Avoid self-"put-downs" or name calling.
- Be willing to give positive and negative feedback to others in respectful ways.
- Be willing to accept feedback from others without becoming verbally or physically aggressive/defensive.
- Maintain confidentiality outside of the group.
- Assist the group in developing any additional rules of its own.

Step 3: Introduce Clients to the Stages of Change

Distribute the "Stages of Change" handout (P/C/P-1.1) and draw a stage diagram on a chalkboard/flipchart to introduce the clients to the stages. (Suggest that, as you describe each stage, they think about a behavior that they have successfully changed on their own and remember how they went through the various stages.)

- Precontemplation. The *precontemplation* stage is one in which individuals are either unconvinced that they have a problem or are unwilling to consider change.
- Contemplation. The *contemplation* stage is one in which a person is actively considering the possibility of change. People in this stage are evaluating options but are not ready to take action at present.
- Preparation. In the *preparation* stage, individuals make a commitment as well as initial plans to change the behavior.
- Action. Once people take effective action to make the change, they are considered to be in the *action* stage. In action, a person adopts strategies to prevent a relapse and a return to the problem behavior.
- Maintenance. The *maintenance* stage of change is one in which the individual consolidates the change and integrates it into his or her lifestyle.

Explain that everyone goes through these stages as they are attempting to change behavior. However, it is also natural for people to "recycle" through (i.e., revisit) earlier stages several times before successfully making and maintaining the change. Explain that rather than being viewed as a failure, a "slip" can be seen as an opportunity to provide useful information and experiences for the next attempt.

Step 4: Conduct a Staging Exercise

Read the following vignettes aloud one at a time. After each scenario, ask group members which stage of change they think applies. Give "hints" as needed, and refer to the staging diagram on the chalkboard/flipchart. Remind clients that they can refer to their "Stages of Change" handout (P/C/P-1.1) as well.

Staging Vignettes

Joseph has been thinking about losing weight, but he just hasn't been able to start exercising like he used to. He has done sit-ups a few mornings during the last several weeks, and he has pumped up the tires on his bicycle. He has also talked to some of his friends who lift weights to see what their routines are. After lunch today, though, he took a nap instead of working out like he had planned. [Preparation]

Jane gets tired of everyone nagging at her to stop smoking. "Why don't they just leave me alone?" she says. It's bad enough that they raised the price of cigarettes this year, and now she can't even smoke in her office during the day. While she's outside on her break she thinks, "I can't get any work done without a cigarette. How do they expect me to finish this project on time if I have to keep coming outside to think?" [Precontemplation]

Marcus is proud of himself. He has gone for 2 weeks without taking a drink. He has started "hanging out" with some new friends at work who don't drink either, and his work has improved; his boss even noticed a difference! When he threw out all the alcohol from his house a few weeks ago, he wasn't sure his resolve would last. Even though he's been tempted to stop by the bar during "happy hour" after work, he has instead jogged in the park every evening. [Action]

Maria wonders if all this stuff about how caffeine can hurt your baby is true. She has been drinking five cups of coffee a day for as long as she can remember, and it hasn't seemed to do anything to her before. Still, she hasn't been able to sleep since she became pregnant, and now her stomach gets upset after even one cup of coffee. She saw some babies at the hospital that were really tiny, and the doctor says it's due to caffeine. "Maybe I should consider cutting down a little," she thinks. [Contemplation]

It's hard for Paul to believe it's been over 2 years since he used cocaine. The kids at the shelter where he volunteers remind him of himself at that age—it doesn't seem like so long ago he was addicted to crack himself. It hasn't been easy to stay clean, but it sure has been worth it. He recently told someone that it's nice to go to sleep at night without hating himself and everyone else. [Maintenance]

Step 5: Determine Clients' Stages of Change

Distribute the "Where Am I?" handout (P/C/P-1.2). Demonstrate how to determine stage for any kind of change by using the cues on the handout. As an example, we suggest that you choose a nonthreatening behavior such as diet or exercise. Explain that a person can be in different stages of change for various behaviors. For example, someone might be in the contemplation stage for quitting smoking but in the action stage for losing weight. Next, instruct clients to think about their primary substance of abuse; have them read the cues and decide which stage they are in for that substance. Assist clients as needed. Facilitate a group discussion about clients' reactions to this exercise. Remember to avoid argumentation, express empathy, roll with resistance, and support clients' confidence in their ability to change.

Some suggestions to prompt discussion are as follows:

- Were you able to identify your stage of change?
- Can you see how you might be in another stage for a different behavior?
- Can you describe an experience where you were at one stage and went back to an earlier stage?
- Can you share an experience where you moved through all the stages and are now in maintenance for a behavior?

Step 6: Close the Session

As a transition to closing the session, check in with group members to see if anyone has additional issues he or she wants to discuss before the session ends. At the close of each session, summarize what has occurred in the group that day. Ask clients if you have missed anything, or if they would like to add anything to your summary. Stress that this group is intended to help members move through the stages of change, and the facilitator is available to assist in helping to deal with drug or alcohol problems. However, the decision of whether to change is up to each individual. No one will "force" them to do anything; the responsibility for change is theirs.

STEP-BY-STEP SESSION TASKS

Step 1: Open the session (approximately 10 minutes).

- Briefly introduce yourself to the group.
- Introduce the motivational approach.
- Have group members introduce themselves and tell one thing they would like to get out of the group.

Step 2: Establish group rules (approximately 10 minutes).

- Facilitate discussion about the motivational approach.
- Assist clients in developing group rules.

Step 3: Introduce clients to the stages of change (approximately 15 minutes).

- Distribute the "Stages of Change" handout (P/C/P-1.1).
- Draw a stage diagram on a chalkboard/flipchart and explain stages.
- Emphasize that people cycle through the stages, and that a "slip" does not mean failure.

Step 4: Conduct a staging exercise (approximately 10 minutes).

- Read vignettes aloud one at a time (see "Implementation").
- Have clients guess which stage of change applies to each vignette after it is read.
- Refer to the staging diagram on the chalkboard/flipchart as you discuss each scenario.

Step 5: Determine clients' stages of change (approximately 20 minutes).

- Distribute the "Where Am I?" handout (P/C/P-1.2).
- Demonstrate how to determine stage, using an example of a nonthreatening problem behavior.
- Assist group members in determining their own stages of change.
- Facilitate a group discussion about this activity.

Step 6: Close the session (approximately 10 minutes).

- Summarize the session.
- Check in with group members.

STAGES OF CHANGE

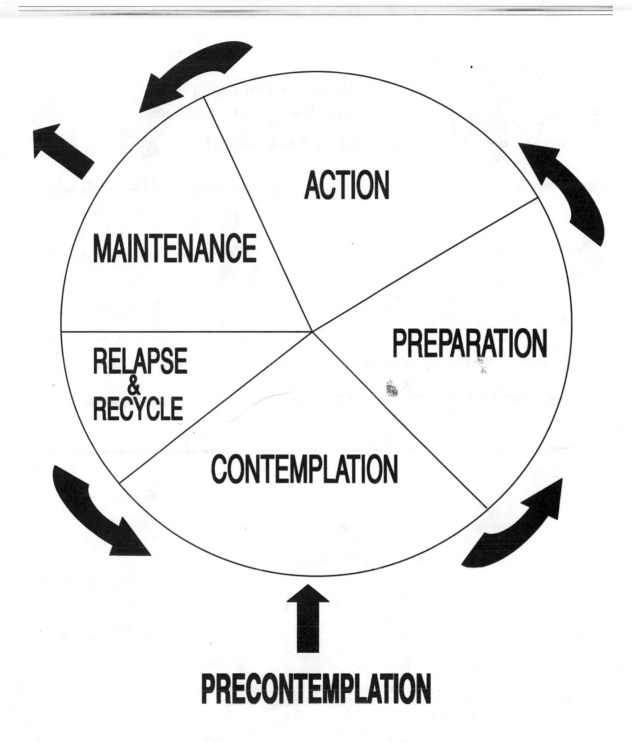

WHERE AM I?

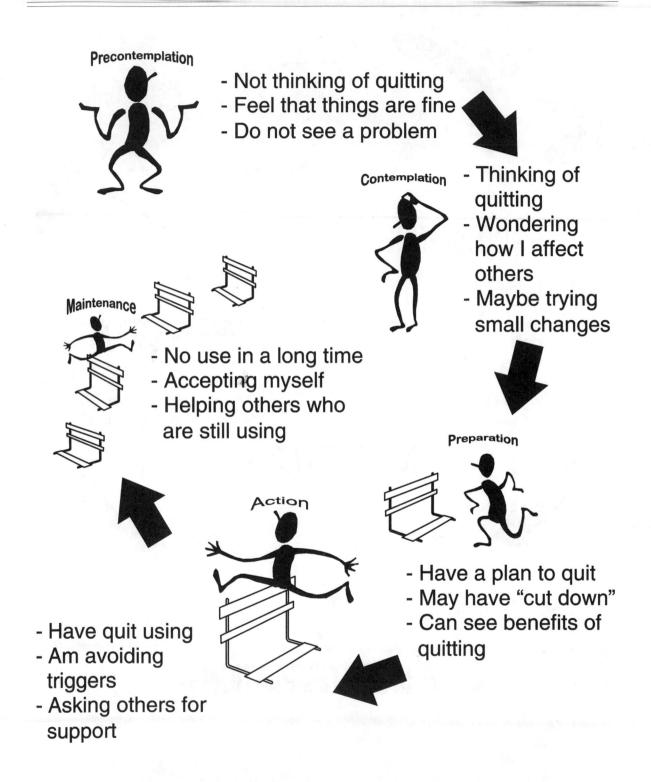

Precontemplation
- Not thinking of quitting
- Feel that things are fine
- Do not see a problem

Contemplation
- Thinking of quitting
- Wondering how I affect others
- Maybe trying small changes

Maintenance
- No use in a long time
- Accepting myself
- Helping others who are still using

Preparation
- Have a plan to quit
- May have "cut down"
- Can see benefits of quitting

Action
- Have quit using
- Am avoiding triggers
- Asking others for support

P/C/P SESSION 2

A Day in the Life

RATIONALE

Consciousness raising involves increasing knowledge about oneself or the nature of one's problem. This session helps *raise* clients' *consciousness* about the quantity and frequency of their substance use. Clients in the early stages of change are often unaware of exactly how much and how often they are using. By asking clients to describe a usual or "typical" day, we can elicit this information from them in a nonthreatening manner.

CONTENT OBJECTIVES

Increase client awareness of the quantity and frequency of substance use.
Increase client awareness of patterns of substance use.

MATERIALS REQUIRED

Copies of the "A Day in the Life" handout (P/C/P-2.1) for distribution to each group member

SESSION SUMMARY

The facilitator explains that sometimes it can be difficult for people to realize how much and how often they are using alcohol or other drugs. Clients are asked to write their answers to the questions on the handout "A Day in the Life" (P/C/P-2.1). This

47

asks them to describe their typical pattern of substance use throughout a single day. No one will collect the handouts, and clients do not need to reveal anything they choose not to. Group members discuss both what they have learned about their own use through this exercise and the times during the year that their substance use might be more or less than the usual amount (such as birthdays, holidays, weekends, and so on).

IMPLEMENTATION

Sometimes it can be difficult for clients to realize how much or how often they are using alcohol or other drugs. Dr. Stephen Rollnick and colleagues (1999) suggest that it can be informative for clients to describe an entire day of use to another person. By detailing their substance use during different parts of the day, they often learn that they are using even more than they realized. This is a nonthreatening way to raise clients' consciousness about the quantity and frequency of their use. An additional step is to have clients think about how their substance might differ during specific times of the year or during special occasions (such as birthdays or family get-togethers). This technique was developed by Drs. Linda and Mark Sobell (1992) in an instrument called the "Timeline Followback."

Steps 1 and 2: Open the Session and Introduce the Topic

Briefly "check in" with the clients to see if there are any remaining issues from the previous session and "touch base" to see how they have been since the previous session.

After checking in with the clients, explain that people who use alcohol or other drugs are not always aware of the frequency and amount of their use. Explain that people often have "patterns" of use. For example, they may have a typical pattern of use during the week and a different pattern on the weekends. Ask clients to spend a few minutes thinking about their use on various days of the week.

Step 3: Describe a Day of Substance Use

Distribute the "A Day in the Life" handout (P/C/P-2.1) and read the instructions aloud. The clients are to write down descriptions of their substance use on the handout to learn as much as they can about their use during a *typical* day (i.e., those days that represent their most usual pattern). The questions on the handout encourage clients to describe their use during specific parts of their day. Read the first question aloud: "Let's start with the morning. Describe your use from the time you wake up in the morning until around noon." Allow clients to think about this for a few minutes and write their responses; circulate among the group and offer assistance. Repeat this procedure with the remaining two questions. If clients have trouble identifying a "typical" day, ask them to focus on a recent day of drinking or drug use.

Step 4: Discuss the Activity

Ask clients to share what they may have learned about their substance use through this exercise. Facilitate a group discussion by saying something like "Now that you've looked at your substance use for a typical day, think about times when you might drink or use differently." Some questions to prompt their thoughts are as follows:

- "Do you tend to drink/use more or less than your usual amount on *weekends*?"
- "Are there specific *occasions* when you might drink/use more or less than your usual amount [such as birthdays, family get-togethers, and so on]?"
- "Are there times during *each month* that you might drink or use more or less than the usual amount [such as holidays or pay-days]?"

Step 5: Close the Session

Briefly check in with the group to see if clients have any further questions or concerns, and summarize the session.

STEP-BY-STEP SESSION TASKS

Step 1: Open the session and check in with the group (approximately 10 minutes).

Step 2: Introduce the topic: A day in the life (approximately 5 minutes).

- Explain that people who use alcohol or other drugs often are unaware of how much and how often they use.
- Point out that people tend to drink or use drugs in "patterns" (i.e., they have typical amounts and times that they usually use).

Step 3: Describe a typical day of substance use (approximately 20 minutes).

- Distribute the "A Day in the Life" handout (P/C/P-2.1) to each group member.
- Read and explain the instructions.
- Read the first question on the handout aloud ("Let's start with the morning. Describe your use from the time you wake up in the morning until around noon").
- Allow clients to think about this for a few minutes and write their responses; circulate among the group and offer assistance.
- Repeat this with the remaining two questions on the handout.

Step 4: Discuss this activity (approximately 10 minutes)

- Ask clients to share what they may have learned about their substance use through this exercise.

- Facilitate a group discussion, asking clients to think about times that their drinking or drug use might be different from their typical use (during weekends, anniversaries, holidays, paydays, and so on).

Step 5: Close the session (approximately 5 minutes).

- Briefly check in with the group.
- Summarize the session.

A DAY IN THE LIFE

Describe your day in terms of your alcohol *and* other drug use. It might be helpful to pick a "typical" day—one that gives the best example of your use.

Let's start with the morning. Describe your use from the time you wake up in the morning until around noon.

Now, how about your use from noon until early evening, say around 6 P.M.? Please describe.

Finally, describe your substance use from around 6 P.M., or suppertime, until you go to bed at night.

Physiological Effects of Alcohol

CHANGE PROCESS OBJECTIVE: CONSCIOUSNESS RAISING

RATIONALE

Consciousness raising involves increasing knowledge about oneself and the nature of the problem behavior. This session helps *raise* clients' *consciousness* about the extent of their *alcohol* use and helps them to identify problems associated with their use. By completing and self-scoring the Alcohol Use Disorders Identification Test (AUDIT), clients learn about their level of risk. This session also educates clients about the physiological effects of alcohol and how it may affect their health.

CONTENT OBJECTIVES

Clients complete a brief exercise to determine extent of alcohol use.
Clients learn various ways that alcohol can harm the body physiologically.

MATERIALS REQUIRED

Copies of the following for distribution to each group member:
Alcohol Use Disorders Identification Test (AUDIT) handout (P/C/P-3.1)
"Scoring the AUDIT" handout (P/C/P-3.2)
"AUDIT—What Does It Mean?" handout (P/C/P-3.3)
"What Can Alcohol Do?" handout (P/C/P-3.4)
Pens/pencils

SESSION SUMMARY

In today's session, clients will complete the "Alcohol Use Disorders Identification Test (AUDIT)" and score their own assessments. Clients are not asked to reveal their scores, but a group discussion is held in which the norms (or "average") scores and their meanings are presented. The facilitator then presents information from the National Institute on Alcohol Abuse and Alcoholism regarding the physiological effects of alcohol. See the "Implementation" section for how to carry out these tasks using a motivational approach.

IMPLEMENTATION

Some clients may be unaware of their level of alcohol consumption and the personal and social harm their drinking is causing them. There are two goals for this session: (1) for clients to learn more about their level of alcohol use and consequences through completion of a standardized assessment tool; and (2) to raise clients' consciousness about the potentially harmful effects of alcohol use.

Many times, clients hold the belief that "this could never happen to *me*," insisting that they are somehow exempt from physical consequences of their drinking. Another common response sounds something like "I've been drinking for years and have never been sick because of it." Trying to *debate* these arguments with the clients is often counterproductive—remember that the goal of this session is not to convince everyone that drinking can be "bad for them"; you are simply providing information to make them more aware of how alcohol has affected the majority of people who abuse.

A word of caution. Be careful to avoid raising defensiveness in clients during this session. Instead of reading the information about the physiological effects of alcohol *verbatim*, try to highlight the main points; reading the entire handout could cause you to seem "preachy" or judgmental. While we want to give clients the information, we want to do so in a motivational way. Strongly encourage clients to read this handout on their own (or with a friend) after the session.

Steps 1 and 2: Open the Session and Introduce the Topic

After briefly checking in with the group, explain that in today's session you will be talking about alcohol use and that you will be talking about other drug use in a future session. Explain that it is often useful for people to have an opportunity to do some "self-assessment." This is a private way of getting feedback about the level of use and the consequences surrounding that use. Tell clients that they will be completing the Alcohol Use Disorders Identification Test, which is known as the AUDIT. It is a short questionnaire that is often used to provide information about a person's drinking. Assure them that no one will collect the handouts, and they will not be asked to reveal their scores.

Step 3: Complete and Score the AUDIT

Distribute the "Alcohol Use Disorders Identification Test (AUDIT)" handout (P/C/P-3.1), and read the instructions aloud. Stress that clients are to circle only *one* answer per question. Then, read each question aloud, giving clients time to mark their answers on the handout. When they have finished, distribute the "Scoring the AUDIT" handout (P/C/P-3.2). Read each question aloud again, and have clients write the number that corresponds to their answer on the blank line next to each question. Have clients total these numbers; walk among them to help as needed.

Step 4: Interpret AUDIT Results

When everyone has completed the addition, distribute the "AUDIT—What Does It Mean?" handout (P/C/P-3.3). Read each scoring range aloud, summarizing what each represents. Facilitate a discussion about how these scores can be helpful in pointing out how much alcohol clients are currently using and some possible consequences that might occur as a result of continued drinking.

Step 5: Discuss Potential Physiological Effects of Alcohol

Explain that people with high scores on the AUDIT are often at risk for physical complications as a result of their drinking. Distribute the "What Can Alcohol Do?" handout (P/C/P-3.4) and briefly go through each section, asking if any of the group members have known anyone who has had physical problems that sound similar to those listed. (Be sure to put the information in informal terms, paraphrasing and using your own words, rather than sounding "preachy" or "teachy.")

Step 6: Close the Session

Briefly check in with the group and summarize the session by pointing out that you have covered quite a bit of information in today's session. Emphasize that it would be helpful for clients to review each of the handouts before the next session and to bring any questions that they might have to the next group.

STEP-BY-STEP SESSION TASKS

Step 1: Open the session and check in with the group (approximately 10 minutes).

Step 2: Introduce the topic: Physiological effects of alcohol (approximately 10 minutes).

- Explain to clients that in today's session you will be talking about alcohol use specifically and that you will be talking about other drug use in a future session.

- Explain that it is often useful to people to have an opportunity to do some "self-assessment."
- Tell clients that they will be completing the AUDIT (a short questionnaire that is often used to provide information about a person's drinking).
- Tell clients that their answers and score are private.

Step 3: Complete and score the AUDIT (approximately 15 minutes).

- Distribute the "Alcohol Use Disorders Identification Test (AUDIT)" handout (P/C/P-3.1), and read the instructions aloud.
- Stress that clients are to circle only *one* answer per question.
- Read each question aloud, giving clients time to mark their answers on the handout.
- Distribute the "Scoring the AUDIT" handout (P/C/P-3.2).
- Read each question aloud again, and have clients write the number that corresponds to their answer on the blank line next to each question.
- Have the clients total these numbers; walk among them to help with addition as needed.

Step 4: Interpret AUDIT results (approximately 10 minutes).

- Distribute the "AUDIT—What Does It Mean?" handout (P/C/P-3.3).
- Read each scoring range aloud, summarizing what each one represents.
- Facilitate a discussion about these scores.

Step 5: Discuss potential physiological effects of alcohol (approximately 10 minutes).

- Explain that people who score high on the AUDIT are often at risk for physical and other complications as a result of their drinking.
- Distribute the "What Can Alcohol Do?" handout (P/C/P-3.4).
- Briefly read each section, asking if any of the group members have known anyone who has had physical problems that sound similar to those listed.
- Be sure to put the information in informal terms by paraphrasing.

Step 6: Close the session (approximately 5 minutes).

- Briefly check-in with the group.
- Summarize the session.
- Explain that you have covered quite a bit of information during this session, and that it would be helpful to review the materials before the next session.

ALCOHOL USE DISORDERS IDENTIFICATION TEST (AUDIT)

Please circle one answer for each question about your use of alcohol prior to entering this group. (One drink is equal to one can, glass, or bottle of beer, one shot of liquor or one mixed drink, or one glass of wine.)

1. In the past 3 months before entering this program, how often did you have a drink containing alcohol?

    | Never | Monthly or less | Two to four times a month | Two to three times a week | Four or more times a week |

2. In the past 3 months before entering this program, how many drinks containing alcohol did you have on a typical day when drinking?

    | 1 or 2 | 3 or 4 | 5 or 6 | 7 to 9 | 10 or more |

3. In the past 3 months before entering this program, how often did you have six or more drinks on one occasion?

    | Never | Less than monthly | Monthly | Weekly | Daily or almost daily |

4. How often during the last year have you found that you were not able to stop drinking once you had started?

    | Never | Less than monthly | Monthly | Weekly | Daily or almost daily |

5. How often during the last year have you failed to do what was normally expected from you because of drinking?

    | Never | Less than monthly | Monthly | Weekly | Daily or almost daily |

6. How often during the last year have you needed a drink first thing in the morning to get yourself going after a heavy drinking session?

    | Never | Less than monthly | Monthly | Weekly | Daily or almost daily |

7. How often during the last year have you had a feeling of guilt or remorse after drinking?

    | Never | Less than monthly | Monthly | Weekly | Daily or almost daily |

8. How often during the last year have you been unable to remember what happened the night before because you had been drinking?

    | Never | Less than monthly | Monthly | Weekly | Daily or almost daily |

9. Have you or someone else been injured as a result of your drinking?

    | No | Yes, but not in the last year | Yes, during the last year |

10. Has a relative or friend, or a doctor or other health worker, been concerned about your drinking or suggested you cut down?

    | No | Yes, but not in the last year | Yes, during the last year |

SCORING THE AUDIT

For each answer that you circled, write the corresponding number on the line to the right of the question. Then, add those numbers to get a "Total" at the bottom of the page.

1. In the past 3 months before entering this program, how often did you have a drink containing alcohol?

Never	Monthly or less	Two to four times a month	Two to three times a week	Four or more times a week
0	1	2	3	4	_____

2. In the past 3 months before entering this program, how many drinks containing alcohol did you have on a typical day when drinking?

1 or 2	3 or 4	5 or 6	7 to 9	10 or more
0	1	2	3	4	_____

3. In the past 3 months before entering this program, how often did you have six or more drinks on one occasion?

Never	Less than monthly	Monthly	Weekly	Daily or almost daily
0	1	2	3	4	_____

4. How often during the last year have you found that you were not able to stop drinking once you had started?

Never	Less than monthly	Monthly	Weekly	Daily or almost daily
0	1	2	3	4	_____

5. How often during the last year have you failed to do what was normally expected from you because of drinking?

Never	Less than monthly	Monthly	Weekly	Daily or almost daily
0	1	2	3	4	_____

6. How often during the last year have you needed a drink first thing in the morning to get yourself going after a heavy drinking session?

Never	Less than monthly	Monthly	Weekly	Daily or almost daily
0	1	2	3	4	_____

7. How often during the last year have you had a feeling of guilt or remorse after drinking?

Never	Less than monthly	Monthly	Weekly	Daily or almost daily
0	1	2	3	4	_____

8. How often during the last year have you been unable to remember what happened the night before because you had been drinking?

Never	Less than monthly	Monthly	Weekly	Daily or almost daily
0	1	2	3	4	_____

9. Have you or someone else been injured as a result of your drinking?

No	Yes, but not in the last year	Yes, during the last year
0	2	4	_____

10. Has a relative or friend, or a doctor or other health worker, been concerned about your drinking or suggested you cut down?

No	Yes, but not in the last year	Yes, during the last year
0	2	4	_____

TOTAL: _____

AUDIT—WHAT DOES IT MEAN?

The AUDIT is often used as a way of learning important information about drinking in a short period of time. By asking questions about the amount of drinking in the last year, and about things that sometimes happen when people begin drinking heavily, the AUDIT can help you "find out" if your drinking is reaching a dangerous level.

This is what the scores on the AUDIT mean:

If your score is between **1** and **7** make a check mark on this line: _____
- A score in this range indicates that your drinking has not yet reached a dangerous level. You may have a few drinks each week, and drinking may not have begun to cause trouble with other people in your life. If you have a score toward the high end of this range (like 6 or 7), you might want to start paying more attention to how much you are drinking, and how this may be affecting other people in your life.

If your score is between **8** and **20** make a check mark on this line: _____
- A score in this range indicates that your drinking has now reached a *harmful* and *hazardous* level. You may be drinking every day, having blackouts (where you can't remember the night before), and feeling guilt or remorse after drinking. Once you start drinking, it may be difficult for you to stop, and you may be having trouble following through on your responsibilities because of your drinking. You may have even hurt someone in your life as a result of your drinking.

If your score is between **21** and **40** make a check mark on this line: _____
- A score in this range indicates that your drinking has now reached a *very dangerous* level. Almost all the questions on the AUDIT probably sound very familiar to you. There may be days when you cannot even get out of bed because of your drinking, and you may have trouble thinking about anything else. You may be experiencing many physical problems as a result of your heavy drinking.

WHAT CAN ALCOHOL DO?

According to the National Institute on Alcohol Abuse and Alcoholism (Miller, Zweben, DiClemente, & Rychtarik, 1995; NIAAA, 1999), there are many ways that alcohol can affect your body:

- Heart disease—Some heavy drinkers can develop heart trouble because alcohol can weaken the muscles in and around the heart. Also, heavy drinking can lead to high blood pressure, heart disease, hypertension, and increased risk for some kinds of stroke.

- Brain—Alcoholism may "speed up" normal aging or cause premature aging of the brain. Research also shows that shrinkage of the frontal lobes increases with heavy drinking and is related to intellectual impairment in both older and younger drinkers.

- Digestive problems—Heavy drinkers are more prone to have excessive heartburn, ulcers, and even bleeding in the digestive system. They may suffer from illnesses caused by an injured pancreas as well. The pancreas helps to regulate the amount of blood sugar by making insulin. When there is heavy drinking, the pancreas can be affected by becoming inflamed and extremely painful. This is called "pancreatitis" and it can cause diabetes or even death. Symptoms of pancreatitis are severe abdominal pain and excessive weight loss.

  Also, drinking alcohol interferes with sugar processing and the hormones that regulate sugar levels. Chronic heavy drinkers often have low levels of healthy blood sugars (called glucose). Because many heavy drinkers go without proper food while they are drinking, their stores of healthy sugar can be exhausted in a few hours. Also, the body's monitoring of sugar can be affected while alcohol is being digested. The combination of these effects can cause severely low levels of blood sugar (a condition called "hypoglycemia") from 6 to 36 hours after a binge-drinking episode. Failure to treat this condition could have life-threatening results.

- Alcohol-related liver disease—Some drinkers develop alcoholic hepatitis, or inflammation of the liver, as a result of heavy drinking. Symptoms include fever; yellowing of the skin, eyeballs, and urine ("jaundice"); and pain in the abdomen. Although this condition can cause death if alcohol consumption continues, the process can be reversed. Another way that alcohol can affect the liver is by causing "cirrhosis"—10 to 20% of all heavy drinkers develop this disease. This scarring of the liver prevents it from filtering out the waste from the body and can cause death. Unlike alcoholic hepatitis, it is not possible to reverse the damage done to the liver by cirrhosis, although the symptoms can be relieved and liver functioning can improve by abstaining from alcohol. Treatment for the complications caused by cirrhosis is available, and the last resort is liver transplantation. However, alcohol-induced liver damage can disrupt the body's metabolism, eventually impairing the function of other organs.

- Cancer—Long-term heavy drinking increases the risk of developing several types of cancer because alcohol reduces the body's ability to fight diseases and infections. Some forms of cancer

(continued)

are especially common in heavy drinkers such as cancer of the esophagus, mouth, throat, and voice box. Women who drink two or more drinks a day are at greater risk of developing breast cancer. Other cancers that may be related to heavy drinking include cancer of the colon and the rectum.

• Reproductive system—Heavy drinking has a major effect on the reproductive system, affecting sex drive, fertility, and pregnancy. For instance, alcohol is directly harmful to the testes, causing reduced testosterone levels in men. Prolonged low testosterone levels may contribute to a "femininization" of male sexual characteristics, for example, breast enlargement. In women, chronic heavy drinking can contribute to numerous reproductive disorders, including cessation of or irregular menstruation, menstrual cycles without ovulation, early menopause, and increased risk of spontaneous abortions. Drinking during pregnancy can have numerous harmful effects on the fetus, such as disease (fetal alcohol syndrome), miscarriages, birth defects, and mental retardation. Finally, alcohol dependence and related medical problems, such as brain and liver damage, tend to progress more rapidly in women than in men.

• Breathing disorders—People who drink heavily appear to be at increased risk for sleep apnea, especially if they snore. Sleep apnea is a condition where the upper air passage narrows or closes during sleep, resulting in a lack of oxygen to the brain. In addition, drinking alcohol at night can lead to narrowing of the air passage, causing episodes of apnea. Alcohol's depressant effects can increase the duration of periods of apnea as well. Among patients with severe sleep apnea, heavy drinking is associated with five times the risk for fatigue-related traffic accidents compared to people with apnea who do not drink alcohol. Finally, the combination of alcohol, sleep apnea, and snoring increases a person's risk for heart attack, arrhythmia, stroke, and sudden death.

Physiological Effects of Drugs

CHANGE PROCESS OBJECTIVE: CONSCIOUSNESS RAISING

RATIONALE

Consciousness raising involves clients' increasing knowledge about themselves and the nature of the problem behavior. This session helps clients to become aware of the extent of their drug use and to identify problems associated with their use. By completing and self-scoring a drug screening instrument, clients learn about their level of risk. This session also educates clients about the physiological effects of drugs and how they may affect their health.

CONTENT OBJECTIVES

Clients complete a brief exercise to determine extent of drug use.
Clients learn various ways that drugs can harm the body physiologically.

MATERIALS REQUIRED

Copies of the following for distribution to each group member:
"Drug Screening Inventory" handout (P/C/P-4.1)
"Scoring the Drug Screening Inventory" handout (P/C/P-4.2)
"What Can Drugs Do?" handout (P/C/P-4.3)

SESSION SUMMARY

In today's session, clients will complete the Drug Screening Inventory and score their own assessments. Clients are not asked to reveal their scores, but a group discussion is held in which the range of scores and their meanings are presented. The facilitator then presents information from the National Institute on Drug Abuse about the physiological effects of various types of drugs.

IMPLEMENTATION

Clients may be unaware of the extent to which their drug use has negatively affected their lives. In today's session, clients will complete a brief self-assessment tool (Drug Screening Inventory) designed to provide information regarding their drug use. Because there are so many different types of drugs, and each drug can have different effects on the body, we have compiled a summary based upon information from the National Institute on Drug Abuse.

As in the previous session, you may find clients believing that this will "never happen to me," or that they have not had any trouble "so far." Remember to "roll with resistance"! Also, remind the group that you are sharing information for those clients who may not have known the potential harm that drugs can cause on the body.

A word of caution. Be careful to avoid raising defensiveness in clients during this session. Instead of reading the information about the physiological effects of drugs *verbatim*, try to highlight the main points for each drug. Reading the entire handout could cause you to seem "preachy" or judgmental. While we want to give clients the information, we want to do so in a motivational way. Keep in mind that it is not your job to convince clients of the effect their drug use may be having on their lives. We want to provide accurate information (even a little advice is OK) but, ultimately, it is up to the client to decide what, if anything, he or she will do with the information.

Steps 1 and 2: Open the Session and Introduce the Topic

Briefly check in with the group and introduce the topic by reminding clients how useful it can be to have an opportunity to do some "self-assessment." Explain that in today's session they will be completing the Drug Screening Inventory. This is a short questionnaire that is often used to provide information about a person's drug use.

Step 3: Complete and Score the Drug Screening Inventory

[*Note.* The Drug Screening Inventory was developed for the specific purpose of assessing the extent of clients' drug use. This inventory is based on the criteria for substance abuse and dependence found in the fourth edition of the *Diagnostic and Statistical Manual of Mental Disorders* (American Psychiatric Association, 1994). As you will see in the interpretation section below, the scoring mechanism of this inventory allows the facilitator to determine whether clients have been engaging in at risk, abusive, or dependent patterns of use.]

Distribute the "Drug Screening Inventory" handout (P/C/P-4.1) and read the directions to the group. Make sure clients understand that the test refers to drugs that are used nonmedically or in excess of a prescription. Also, have them simply *circle* their answer—ask them not to write anything in the blank at this time. Read each question aloud and have clients circle their answers as you go.

Distribute the "Scoring the Drug Screening Inventory" handout (P/C/P-4.2), and read the instructions found in Part I. Explain that for *questions 1 through 4*, for each "Yes" that clients circled, they should write a "1" on the line to the right of the question, and for each "No," they should write "0." Then, explain that for *questions 5 through 11*, for each "Yes" that they circled, clients should write a "5" on the line to the right of the question, and for each "No," they are to write a "0." Give group members time to score their own assessments, and circulate to offer assistance as needed. After clients have completed this step, have them add the numbers together and write the total on the appropriate line at the bottom of the page; again, circulate among group members to help, as needed.

Step 4: Interpret Drug Screening Results

Read the categories found in Part II of the "Scoring the Drug Screening Inventory" handout (P/C/P-4.2), having clients follow along as you read. Explain the differences between the four levels of use. Facilitate a group discussion about how these scores can be helpful in pointing out the level of drugs clients are currently using, and some possible consequences that might occur as a result of continued drug use.

Step 5: Discuss Potential Physiological Effects of Drugs

Explain that people who score in the two highest levels on the Drug Screening Inventory are often at risk for physical complications as a result of their drug use. Distribute the "What Can Drugs Do?" handout (P/C/P-4.3) and briefly highlight the information for each drug, asking if any of the group members have known anyone who has had physical problems that sound similar to those listed. (Be sure to put the information in informal terms, paraphrasing and using your own words, rather than sounding "preachy").

Step 6: Close the Session

Briefly check in with the group and summarize the session by pointing out that you have covered quite a bit of information in today's session. Thank clients for their participation and willingness to think about their substance use. Tell them that "feedback" is often very helpful for people who are deciding if they might want to make some changes in their lives. Remind them that you will not be pushing them to change but are available to help if they do decide there are any changes they want to make in their lives.

STEP-BY-STEP SESSION TASKS

Step 1: Open the session and check in with the group (approximately 10 minutes).

Step 2: Introduce the topic: Physiological effects of drugs (approximately 5 minutes).

Step 3: Complete and score the Drug Screening Inventory (approximately 15 minutes).

- Distribute the "Drug Screening Inventory" handout (P/C/P-4.1).
- Read the directions to the group.
- Read each question aloud, and have clients circle their answers as you go (they do not need to write anything in the blank at this time).
- Distribute the "Scoring the Drug Screening Inventory" handout (P/C/P-4.2).
- Read the instructions found in Part I.
- Help the group members privately score their own assessments, circulating to offer assistance as needed.
- Have the clients add the numbers together and write the total on the appropriate line at the bottom of the page.
- Circulate among the clients to help with addition, as needed.

Step 4: Interpret Drug Screening results (approximately 10 minutes).

- Read the categories found in Part II of the "Scoring the Drug Screening Inventory" handout (P/C/P-4.2).
- Explain the differences between the four levels of use.
- Facilitate a group discussion about how these scores can be helpful in pointing out how much drugs clients are currently using, and some possible consequences that might occur as a result of continued drug use.

Step 5: Discuss potential physiological effects of drugs (approximately 10 minutes).

- Explain that people who score in the two highest levels on the Drug Screening Inventory are often at risk for physical complications as a result of their drug use.
- Distribute the "What Can Drugs Do?" handout (P/C/P-4.3).
- Briefly highlight the information for each drug, asking if any of the group members have known anyone who has had physical problems that sound similar to those listed.
- Be sure to put the information in informal terms by paraphrasing.

Step 6: Close the session (approximately 10 minutes).

- Briefly check in with the group.

- Summarize the session.
- Thank clients for their participation.
- Remind clients that you will not be pushing them to do anything but are available for support if they do decide there are any changes they would like to make.

DRUG SCREENING INVENTORY

The following questions ask about your drug use (not including alcohol) during the past year. The term "drug use" refers to any and all drugs that you have used for the purpose of getting high, intoxicated, or to feel good. Circle "Yes" or "No" for each question below based on your experiences in the past 12 months.

In past 12 months . . .

1. . . . has your drug use affected your ability to take care of your responsibilities (e.g., affected school/work performance or household duties)? Yes No _____

2. . . . have you used drugs in situations where you could have been physically hurt (e.g., driving under the influence)? Yes No _____

3. . . . has your drug use resulted in problems with the law? Yes No _____

4. . . . have you kept using drugs even though it caused problems with family, friends, or other people? Yes No _____

5. . . . have you had to use larger amounts of a drug to get the same effect as before? Yes No _____

6. . . . have you experienced withdrawal symptoms (such as shakes, DTs, sleeping problems) *or* used drugs to make withdrawal symptoms go away? Yes No _____

7. . . . have you used larger amounts of drugs or for a longer time than you meant to? Yes No _____

8. . . . have you often wanted to cut down on your drug use, *or* tried to cut down and couldn't? Yes No _____

9. . . . have you spent a great deal of time getting, using, or getting over the effects of drugs? Yes No _____

10. . . . have you given up important activities because of drug use (e.g., given up work-related activities, doing things with friends, or hobbies)? Yes No _____

11. . . . have you kept using drugs even though you knew it could make you more physically sick or emotionally upset than usual? Yes No _____

Total: _____

SCORING THE DRUG SCREENING INVENTORY

Part I: For questions **1** through **4**, for each "Yes" that you circled, write a "1" on the line to the right of the question. For each "No" that you circled, write a "0" on the line to the right of the question. For questions **5** through **11**, for each "Yes" that you circled, write a "5" on the line to the right of the question. For each "No" that you circled, write a "0" on the line to the right of the question. Then, add those numbers to get a "Total" at the bottom of the page.

Part II: The following categories describe what various scores on the inventory mean.

0   **No problems reported**—If you scored in this range and are using drugs, your drug use has not yet reached a harmful level. You may want to start paying attention to see if any of the items on the exercise start happening.

1 to 4   **Moderate level (abuse)**—If you scored in this range, you have abused drugs in the past year. Your use has begun to affect different areas of your life, and you may have gotten yourself into dangerous situations when using drugs.

5 to 14   **Substantial level**—If you scored in this range, you are at risk for becoming dependent on drugs. You may have noticed that it is difficult to stop using, or that your drug use has affected your ability to take care of your responsibilities.

15 to 39   **Severe level (dependence)**—If you scored in this range, you have been dependent on drugs this past year. You may be feeling that you have lost control of your drug use, and it may be getting harder to function on a daily basis.

WHAT CAN DRUGS DO?

According to the National Institute on Drug Abuse, there are many ways that drugs can affect your body:

• **Inhalants**—Most inhalants are extremely poisonous to the body's organs. Inhalant use may cause damage in the brain (to "neurons" or connectors), leading not only to the loss of reasoning ability but also to psychological and social problems. Significant damage to the liver and kidneys may also occur. Because they cause irregular heartbeat, some inhalants may cause sudden death. Long-term users of inhalants often lose weight, have nosebleeds, mouth sores, and are often irritable or depressed. Nausea, vomiting, and extreme salivation are common side effects.

• **Tobacco**—People who use tobacco products (such as cigarettes and "dip") risk addiction to nicotine, which can lead to heart disease, lung cancer, emphysema, and cancers of the mouth, just to name a few. Tobacco also decreases stamina, can stain teeth, wrinkles the skin, and can result in chronic halitosis (i.e., bad breath).

• **Marijuana**—Short-term problems caused by marijuana include the impairment of coordination, concentration, and short-term memory. Long-term use may lead to a lack of energy and motivation, and impairment of memory. These effects may linger even after the user stops using the drug. Also, heavy use appears to produce approximately the same lung and cancer risks as smoking five times as much tobacco (i.e., cigarettes). As with tobacco, lung damage and the risk of cancer are significant hazards of marijuana use.

• **Cocaine/crack**—In addition to irritability, mood disturbances, restlessness, paranoia, and auditory hallucinations, cocaine/crack can cause several dangerous physical conditions. It can lead to disturbances in heart rhythm and heart attacks, as well as chest pain or even respiratory failure. In addition, strokes, seizures, and headaches are not uncommon in heavy users.

Cocaine use has been linked to many types of heart disease. Cocaine has been found to trigger chaotic heart rhythms, called ventricular fibrillation; accelerate heartbeat and breathing; and increase blood pressure and body temperature. Physical symptoms may include chest pain, nausea, blurred vision, fever, muscle spasms, convulsions, and coma.

Different ways of doing cocaine can produce different physical harm. Regularly snorting cocaine, for example, can lead to loss of sense of smell, nosebleeds, problems with swallowing, hoarseness, and an overall irritation of the nasal septum, which can lead to a chronically inflamed, runny nose. Ingested cocaine can cause a severe intestinal infection (called "gangrene"), due to reduced blood flow in the digestive tract. And people who inject cocaine may also experience an allergic reaction, either to the drug or to some additive, which can result in death. Because cocaine often causes reduced food intake, many chronic cocaine users lose their appetites and can experience significant weight loss and malnourishment. It is important to note that the mixture of cocaine and alcohol is the most common two-drug combination that results in drug-related death.

- **Methamphetamine**—Methamphetamine can cause many types of cardiovascular problems, including rapid heart rate, irregular heartbeat, increased blood pressure, and irreversible, stroke-producing damage to small blood vessels in the brain. Chronic methamphetamine abuse can also result in inflammation of the heart lining and, among users who inject the drug, damaged blood vessels and skin abscesses. Psychotic symptoms can sometimes persist for months or years after use has ceased. Also, research indicates that methamphetamine abuse during pregnancy may result in prenatal complications, increased rates of premature delivery, and altered neonatal behavioral patterns, such as abnormal reflexes and extreme irritability.

- **Heroin**—Chronic heroin abuse can result in scarred and/or collapsed veins, bacterial infections of the blood vessels and heart valves, abscesses (boils) and other soft-tissue infections, and liver or kidney disease. Lung complications (including various types of pneumonia and tuberculosis) may result from the poor health condition of the abuser as well as from heroin's depressing effects on respiration. Sharing needles can lead to some of the most severe consequences of heroin abuse—infections with hepatitis B and C, HIV, and many other blood-borne viruses, which drug abusers can then pass on to their sexual partners and children.

P/C/P SESSION 5

Expectations

CHANGE PROCESS OBJECTIVE: CONSCIOUSNESS RAISING

RATIONALE

Consciousness raising involves clients' increasing knowledge about themselves and the nature of the problem behavior. By identifying and verbalizing their expectations about their substance use, clients *raise* their *consciousness* about their reasons for using. This awareness often serves to increase clients' motivation to change, because it provides them with knowledge about their reasons for using. As clients become more ready to change, they can then work to change their expectancies or engage in alternative behaviors to achieve the desired effect, or expected outcome.

CONTENT OBJECTIVES

Clients learn about their expectations and beliefs about their substance use.
Clients learn alternative behaviors to achieving the desired outcomes.

MATERIALS REQUIRED

Copies of the "My Expectations about Substance Use" handout (P/C/P-5.1) for distribution to each group member.

SESSION SUMMARY

The facilitator explains the concept of "expectations" and the impact they have on behavior. Clients discuss the effects a person might expect from using alcohol and other drugs, then individually complete a brief questionnaire to identify their own expectations. The group discusses alternative behaviors to achieve similar outcomes.

IMPLEMENTATION

People's expectations about certain courses of action can have a powerful effect on their behavior. In the alcohol field, these cognitive factors related to drinking are called "expectancies." They play an important role in people's decision to use, and their consumption levels and drinking patterns. It is helpful for clients to identify both the positive and negative expectancies they have about their substance use.

The questionnaire used in this session, based on the Alcohol Expectancy Questionnaire, originally developed by Dr. Sandy Brown and colleagues in 1980, was among the first to assess alcohol-related expectancies. Subsequently, Dr. Damaris Rohsenow developed the Alcohol Effects Questionnaire (1983), a brief measure that assesses both the positive and negative effects people expect alcohol to have on them.

In this session, we extend this idea of expectancies to include substances other than alcohol. Remember that different substances affect the body and mood in different ways. Cocaine is considered a stimulant, while alcohol acts as both a depressant and a stimulant. Thus, the expectations for using alcohol might differ from expectations for heroin. While we have taken a bit of free license in extending this concept to other substances, we have found that it facilitates a lively and useful session that clients find quite *consciousness raising.*

Steps 1 and 2: Open the Session and Introduce the Topic

Briefly check in with the group and introduce the topic by explaining that people have expectations about certain courses of action, and that these expectations can have a powerful effect on their behavior. For example, many people feel that they can only be comfortable in social situations if they are drinking or using drugs. They say that substance use makes them more relaxed so they are better able to communicate with others. Some people believe that drinking will make them better dancers, or that it will help them perform better sexually. Point out that people also have negative expectancies about substance use, such as getting arrested or feeling bad the next morning.

Step 3: Identify Expectations Involving Alcohol and Other Drugs

Distribute the "My Expectations about Substance Use" handout (P/C/P-5.1). Explain that the eight expectations listed are common to many people. Have clients circle "true" or "false" (T or F), depending on whether a particular expectancy is true for them. These items have been adapted from the Alcohol Effects Questionnaire (Rohsenow, 1983); each item represents a domain of personal beliefs about the effects of substance use.

Step 4: Discuss Client Expectations

After group members have completed the handout, facilitate a discussion about their expectancies. Ask clients to think back to their two most recent episodes of substance use. Questions to prompt discussion are as follows: Did their substance use fulfill their expectations? If not, how did it fall short? If so, can they think of alternatives to substance use in that particular situation? This is a good opportunity to listen for self-motivational statements. Be sure to reinforce clients' ideas about alternatives to using by reflecting and summarizing their positive change statements.

Step 5: Close the Session

Briefly check in with the group. Summarize the session by explaining that since clients have now identified and verbalized their expectations, this awareness may help them in the future when they are faced with decisions about substance use. Affirm the work they have done in the session.

STEP-BY-STEP SESSION TASKS

Step 1: Open the session and check in with the group (approximately 10 minutes).

Step 2: Introduce the topic: Expectations (approximately 10 minutes).

- Point out that both positive and negative expectations affect our behaviors.
- Explain that expectations play an important role in a people's decision to use and their consumption level and substance use pattern.
- Give examples of expectations people might have.

Step 3: Identify expectations involving alcohol and other drugs (approximately 20 minutes).

- Distribute the "My Expectations about Substance Use" handout (P/C/P-5.1).
- Have clients circle "true" or "false" (T or F), depending on whether a particular expectation is true for them.

Step 4: Discuss clients' expectations (approximately 15 minutes).

- Have clients think about their responses and their two most recent episodes of substance use.
- Facilitate a discussion about the following:

  1. How their expectations influence their behavior.
  2. Whether they obtained the expected outcomes the last two times they used.

    3. How awareness about their expectations might help them in the future

Step 5: Close the session (approximately 5 minutes).

- Briefly check in with the group.
- Affirm clients' participation.
- Summarize the session.

MY EXPECTATIONS ABOUT SUBSTANCE USE

Circle "T" for true or "F" for false for the following statements:

Using alcohol or other drugs makes me feel less shy.	T	F
I'm more clumsy after drinking or using drugs.	T	F
I'm more romantic when I use alcohol or other drugs.	T	F
Alcohol or other drugs make the future seem brighter to me.	T	F
When I use alcohol or other drugs, it is easier to tell someone off.	T	F
Using alcohol or other drugs makes me feel good.	T	F
I'm more likely to say embarrassing things after drinking or using other drugs.	T	F
Alcohol or other drugs help me sleep better.	T	F

Expressions of Concern

CHANGE PROCESS OBJECTIVES: SELF-REEVALUATION, DRAMATIC RELIEF

RATIONALE

Self-reevaluation involves rethinking the problem behavior and recognizing when and how this behavior conflicts with personal values. *Dramatic relief* involves experiencing and expressing feelings about the problem behavior.

Since clients in this group are in the early stages of change, some of them may not see their drinking or drug use as problematic. It is helpful to explore whether there are other people in clients' lives who have expressed concern about their substance use. By relating these concerns, clients often gain insight into the problems alcohol or other drugs have caused in their lives. This, together with the results of the AUDIT and Drug Screening Inventory from previous sessions, can help clients begin to reevaluate their substance use. Clients often experience dramatic relief (or emotional arousal) when they make the connection between their use and the concerns of others in their lives.

CONTENT OBJECTIVES

Clients discuss the ways in which others have expressed concern about their substance use.

Clients think about whether they have any personal concerns about their use.

MATERIALS REQUIRED

Copies of the "Who Is Concerned?" handout (P/C/P-6.1) for distribution to each group member.

SESSION SUMMARY

In this session, group members relate concerns that others have shared about their substance use. The facilitator encourages a discussion about these expressions of concern and assists clients in identifying any of their own personal concerns.

IMPLEMENTATION

It can be helpful to discuss times when other people in clients' lives have expressed concern about their substance use. By relating these concerns, clients often gain insight into the problems alcohol or other drugs have caused in their lives. Be aware that clients may often see others' comments or complaints about their substance use as nagging or disapproval rather than as expressions of concern, for example, the spouse or boss who insists that a client be in treatment for his or her substance use. As the facilitator, you may need to help clients reframe these comments as expressions of concern. Also, remind clients that they are indeed worthy of others' concern, since many of them may not currently feel that way. Ask open-ended questions and use reflective listening to encourage clients to elaborate on their feelings about others' concerns.

Steps 1 and 2: Open the Session and Introduce the Session Topic

Briefly check in with the group. Discuss the fact that other people who care about us often comment or express concern about our behavior. Explain that today, clients will have an opportunity to share how other people in their lives have commented or expressed concern about their substance use, and what impact this feedback has had on them. These expressions can come in many forms: for example, if you suspect that a friend is avoiding you because of your behavior when you are using. While this friend has not openly expressed concern, this could be a subtle message that your substance use is a problem. Other expressions of concern could be more obvious, such a family member or spouse telling you that he or she is worried about you. Yet other expressions can be very blatant, such as a boss threatening to fire you, or a probation officer threatening to revoke your probation.

Step 3: Identify People Who Have Expressed Concern

Distribute the "Who Is Concerned?" handout (P/C/P-6.1). Ask clients to think about people in their lives who have expressed concern about their substance use. Review the handout with the group, providing examples for each question. Allow clients approximately 10 minutes to complete the handout on their own.

Step 4: Facilitate a Group Discussion

When clients have completed the handout, ask them to share their responses with the group. Facilitate a group discussion regarding these expressions of concern, and help clients begin to think about any concerns *they* may have about their own substance use. Questions to prompt discussion might be as follows:

- "How did you feel when others expressed concern about your substance use?"
- "Do you think that any of these concerns are valid?"
- "Has there been any specific event that has caused you to be concerned about your alcohol or other drug use?"

Step 5: Close the Session

Summarize the session and ask clients if they have any new awareness after today's group discussion. Remind clients that when someone expresses concern, even in the form of anger, it can also be an expression of caring. Briefly check in with the group and ask if there is anything else members would add about today's session. Affirm their work in today's session.

STEP-BY-STEP SESSION TASKS

Step 1: Open the session and check in with the group (approximately 10 minutes).

Step 2: Introduce the session topic: Expressions of concern (approximately 10 minutes).

- Discuss the fact that other people who care about us often comment or express concern about our behavior.
- Point out that expressions of concern can come in many forms.
- Explain that in today's session, clients will have an opportunity to share how other people in their lives have expressed concern about their substance use.

Step 3: Identify people who have expressed concern (approximately 15 minutes).

- Distribute the "Who Is Concerned?" handout (P/C/P-6.1).
- Have clients think about people in their lives who have expressed concern about their substance use.
- Review the handout with the group, providing examples for each question.
- Allow clients approximately 10 minutes to complete the handout on their own.

Step 4: Facilitate a group discussion (approximately 10 minutes).

- Ask clients to share their responses with the group.
- Facilitate a group discussion using prompts.
- Help clients begin to think about any concerns *they* may have about their own substance use.

Step 5: Close the session (approximately 10 minutes).

- Summarize the session.
- Ask clients if they have any new awareness after today's session.
- Remind clients that when someone expresses concern, even in the form of anger, it can also be an expression of caring.
- Briefly check in with the group.

WHO IS CONCERNED?

Has anyone ever expressed concern about your substance use? If so, who has been concerned? (List names or initials.)

What particular concerns have these people expressed?

In what ways have they expressed their concerns?

Have you personally ever been concerned about your use?

What particular concerns have you had?

Do you still have any of these concerns?

P/C/P SESSION 7

Values

CHANGE PROCESS OBJECTIVE: SELF-REEVALUATION

RATIONALE

Self-reevaluation involves rethinking the problem behavior and recognizing when and how this behavior conflicts with personal values. By identifying their values and then examining how their substance use conflicts with those values, clients will be using the change process of self-rerevaluation.

CONTENT OBJECTIVES

Help clients identify personal values.

Help clients determine how personal values are discrepant with their substance-using behavior.

MATERIALS REQUIRED

Copies of the "What I Value Most in Life" handout (P/C/P-7.1) for distribution to each group member.

SESSION SUMMARY

In this session, clients discuss the meaning of values and the part their own personal values play in their lives. After identifying these personal values, clients complete an exercise designed to highlight the discrepancy between their values and their substance use.

IMPLEMENTATION

Everyone has things in their lives that they value. For some it might be family or work; for others it might be success or good health. It is important for clients to learn how to identify and articulate their values, and to see how their substance use may be discrepant with those values. Miller and Rollnick (1991) point out that this "dissonance" between clients' present state or behavior and what they value can increase their motivation for change. When clients express these discrepancies, use reflective listening to help clarify and reinforce their thoughts about how their substance use has conflicted with their values.

Steps 1 and 2: Open the Session and Introduce the Session Topic

Begin today's session by checking in with the group and introducing the topic of values. Explain that the things people value can be thought of as being the things that are most important in their lives, the things they hold most dear. Point out that what is highly valued by one person may be of little importance to another. Ask the following questions:

- "What are some things that people value most?" (Examples include good health, family, prosperity, and cultural or religious beliefs.)
- "How does what we value change as we go through life?"
- "What do you consider to be most important in your life?"

Step 3: Identify Personal Values

Distribute the "What I Value Most in Life" handout (P/C/P-7.1) and ask clients to think about those values they consider most important. Have them list those values on the left side of the page. Then instruct them to list any ways in which their substance use has interfered with those values on the right side of the page. For instance, if clients value the relationship they have with their children, they would write that on the left-hand side of the page. If their substance use has ever caused hurt or embarrassment to their children, then they would write this on the right-hand side of the page.

Step 4: Explore Discrepancies between Values and Behavior

Facilitate a group discussion about any discrepancies clients have discovered between their values and their behaviors. To prompt this discussion, describe a situation in which a person who really values his or her job is suspended from work due to coming to work intoxicated. Another example would be to note that some group members say that they most value their families. Ask if clients would be willing to share a time in which their substance use interfered with this relationship. Explore what sorts of reactions and feelings these discrepancies evoke. Use reflective listening as you go around the group and listen to clients' responses (examples of reflective listening techniques can be found in Miller & Rollnick, 1991). This exercise is likely to elicit many self-motivational statements, particularly those of *concern* or *intent to change*. Be sure to reinforce any such statements.

Step 5: Close the Session

Briefly check in with the group and summarize the session. Ask clients to take some time each day to assess whether their behaviors are aligned or discrepant with their values.

STEP-BY-STEP SESSION TASKS

Step 1: Open the session and check in with the group (approximately 10 minutes).

Step 2: Introduce the session topic: Values (approximately 10 minutes).

- Facilitate a group discussion regarding values.
- Help clients identify what they value most.

Step 3: Identify personal values (approximately 15 minutes).

- Distribute the "What I Value Most in Life" handout (P/C/P-7.1).
- Ask clients to think about those values they hold as most important; have them list these values on the left-hand side of the handout.
- Then, instruct them to list any ways in which their substance use has interfered with those things that they value most.
- Give an example of something a person might value and how substance use might have interfered with that value.

Step 4: Explore discrepancies between values and behavior (approximately 15 minutes).

- Facilitate a group discussion about any discrepancies clients have discovered between their values and their behaviors.
- Explore what sorts of reactions and feelings these discrepancies evoke.

Step 5: Close the session (approximately 10 minutes).

- Briefly check in with the group.
- Summarize the session.
- Ask clients to take some time each day to assess whether their behaviors are aligned or discrepant with their values.

WHAT I VALUE MOST IN LIFE

Sometimes our behaviors do not match with what we value most in life. For example, people often find that their drinking or drug use jeopardizes their family relationships or jobs.

On the left-hand side of the paper, write what you value most in life. This might include your children, your job, or even your self-respect. Then, on the right, write down any ways in which your substance use has interfered with that which you value.

What I value most	Ways in which my substance use has interfered with this value

Pros and Cons

CHANGE PROCESS OBJECTIVE: DECISIONAL BALANCE

RATIONALE

Decisional balance involves weighing the pros and cons of a behavior. In this session, clients identify the pros and cons of their substance use, and then assign "weights" to them to help determine the importance of each. In doing so, they begin to see the "whole picture" of their substance use, both the positive and the negative aspects.

CONTENT OBJECTIVES

Clients learn how to identify pros and cons of a behavior.
Clients learn how to assign importance to the pros and cons.

MATERIALS REQUIRED

Copies of the following for distribution to each group member:
"Carolyn's Pros and Cons for Alcohol Use" handout (P/C/P-8.1)
"My Pros and Cons for Substance Use" handout (P/C/P-8.2)

SESSION SUMMARY

The facilitator explains that when thinking about a behavior or making decisions, it can be helpful to consider the "pros" and the "cons" for each choice. The clients complete an exercise in which they list the pros and cons for their substance use and then weigh the importance of each. The facilitator reviews this decisional balancing with a client as an example of how to compare the pros and cons, taking into consideration their respective weights.

IMPLEMENTATION

When people make decisions, they typically weigh the costs and benefits of the change they are considering. Janis and Mann (1977) used the metaphor of a balance scale, or a seesaw on which the client weighs the benefits and costs of the behavior. This "decisional balancing" process is put into practice by clients' evaluation of the pros (or the "good things") and the cons (the "not so good" things) about their substance use. People who have successfully changed addictive behaviors in the past say that this decisional balancing process was a critical one in the resolution of their problem behavior (Sobell et al., 1996).

Research shows that when a person is making a behavior change, a "crossover" of the pros and cons is typically seen in the contemplation stage; that is, in precontemplation, the pros for substance use typically outweigh the cons, and in contemplation, they are balanced, with the number of pros and cons being equal. By the time a person reaches preparation, the balance has shifted and the cons for using typically outweigh the pros (DiClemente, 1991).

In this session, clients quantify their pros and cons by making a list of each and assigning relative weights to indicate which things are the most important to them. Keep in mind that each person will have her or his own unique reasons for changing or for staying the same. What tips the balance may be very different from person to person. Some clients may have difficulty identifying the pros of their use. Remind them that any problem has its positive aspects. If it didn't have benefits, the client would have abandoned it long ago.

Steps 1 and 2: Open the Session and Introduce the Topic

Briefly check in with the group and introduce the topic by explaining that it can helpful to consider the "pros" and the "cons" for each choice when thinking about a behavior or making decisions. For instance, if you were trying to decide whether you should get a dog, you might think not only about the fact that a dog can protect your home (pro), and provide companionship (pro) but also that dog food can get expensive (con) and you may not really have enough space for the animal (con).

Explain that, today, you are going to do a similar exercise that focuses on substance use, called "decisional balancing," and how it is helpful in making well-thought-out decisions. Many people who have successfully changed their alcohol or other drug use report that this process was a very important one for them to do when they were considering change.

Step 3: Practice Identifying Pros and Cons

Distribute the "Carolyn's Pros and Cons for Alcohol Use" handout (P/C/P-8.1) and explain that this is a list of pros and cons. Read the example aloud, explaining that this particular client is considering making a change in her alcohol use. She has written both the pros and cons as she struggles with her decision. By completing this exercise, she is able to see clearly the things she considers "good" and "not so good."

Tell clients that you would like for them to complete a similar exercise for their substance use. Distribute the "My Pros and Cons for Substance Use" handout (P/C/P-8.2). Explain that clients can either pick a particular substance or complete the exercise for their substance use in general. Instruct them to write their pros first, then their cons.

Step 4: Practice Assigning Importance to Pros and Cons

After clients have had time to write down their lists, refer them to Part II of the "Carolyn's Pros and Cons for Alcohol Use" handout (P/C/P-8.1). Explain that once Carolyn completed her pros and cons lists, she then went back and assigned to each item a "weight," on a scale of 1 to 4. In this way, she could assess not only the pros and cons but also the relative importance of each—all of which enter into her decision-making process.

Have clients consider each item they have written on their pros and cons list and ask themselves, "How important is this to me when I am making a decision about substance use?" Tell them to rate the pros and cons on a scale from 1 ("Slightly important") to 4 ("Very important").

Step 5: Weigh the Decisional Balance

Have clients compare their columns of pros and cons. Ask them to think about the length of each list. Does one side have more items than the other? They should also look at the rating of importance that they assigned to each item. Many clients find that they have only one or two things on the left side, but that these are weighted so heavily that they balance a longer list on the right side. Explain that one way to think clearly about substance use is to weigh the pros and cons by taking into account the relative importance of each.

Ask for a volunteer to share his or her list of pros and cons and the weights assigned to each, starting with the pros. It can be very helpful for clients to clarify and state their attraction to substances openly, since they are seldom given a chance to examine what they like about their substance use. Also, starting with the pros often leads clients to spontaneously discuss the cons. The facilitator should listen to clients' ambivalence, empathetically reflecting both their pros and cons. (It is important that you not appear to be judging the responses.) Listen carefully when clients express ambivalence and reflect this back to them by summarizing when they have finished. If time permits, review the pros and cons for all clients who are willing to share. This can be a very powerful tool and does not take a great deal of time.

Step 6: Close the Session

Briefly check in with the group and summarize the session by emphasizing that the pros and cons for any behavior, including substance use, tend to vary with time. Their respective weights tend to change as well. Many things can prompt these differences, including relationships, surroundings, and changes in values or beliefs. Point out that it can be helpful (and interesting) for clients to "revisit" decisional balance activities for various behaviors after time has passed. Suggest that they do so at a later date for their substance use.

STEP-BY-STEP SESSION TASKS

Step 1: Open the session and check in with the group (approximately 10 minutes).

Step 2: Introduce the topic: Pros and cons (approximately 10 minutes).

- Explain the concept of weighing pros and cons.
- Give an example of weighing the pros and cons.
- Point out that many people who have made changes in their substance use report that decisional balancing plays an important role in behavior change.

Step 3: Practice identifying pros and cons (approximately 10 minutes).

- Distribute the "Carolyn's Pros and Cons for Alcohol Use" handout (P/C/P-8.1).
- Read and explain how Carolyn listed her pros and cons.
- Distribute the "My Pros and Cons for Substance Use" handout (P/C/P-8.2).
- Have clients generate a pros and cons list for either a particular substance or for their substance use in general.

Step 4: Practice assigning importance to pros and cons (approximately 10 minutes).

- Refer clients back to Carolyn's example.
- Explain how she "weighted" each pro and con.
- Have clients assign weights to their own pros and cons lists on the "My Pros and Cons for Substance Use" handout (P/C/P-8.2).

Step 5: Weigh the decisional balance (approximately 15 minutes).

- Have clients look at the length of each column (i.e., compare the pros and the cons).
- Ask clients to notice the weights they have assigned the pros and cons.
- Explain that by comparing pros and cons, taking their weights into consider-

ation, clients can think more clearly about whether they want to make changes.

- Ask for a volunteer to describe his or her exercise.
- Reflect back the client's ambivalence.

Step 6: Close the session (approximately 5 minutes).

- Briefly check in with the group.
- Summarize the session.
- Explain that the pros and cons (and their weights) can vary across time, and that it can be interesting to "revisit" decisional balance activities for behaviors after time has passed.
- Suggest that the clients redo today's exercise at a later date.

CAROLYN'S PROS AND CONS FOR ALCOHOL USE

PART I: IDENTIFYING THE PROS AND CONS

Pros (The Good Things about My Drinking)	Cons (The Not So Good Things about My Drinking)
It relaxes me.	I'll feel bad the next day.
It helps me avoid thinking about my problems.	I don't take good care of my children when I'm drunk.
It's a way to socialize with my friends.	It's expensive.
It's a way to relieve boredom.	I could hurt someone if I drive when I've been drinking.

PART II: ASSIGNING IMPORTANCE TO THE PROS AND CONS

How important is each item to you in making a decision about your substance use? (Put a rating next to each item.)

1 = Slightly important
2 = Moderately important
3 = Very important
4 = Extremely important

	Pros (The Good Things about My Drinking)		Cons (The Not So Good Things about My Drinking)
2	It relaxes me.	1	I'll feel bad the next day.
4	It helps me avoid thinking about my problems.	4	I don't take good care of my children when I'm drunk.
1	It's a way to socialize with my friends.	3	It's expensive.
1	It's a way to relieve boredom.	4	I could hurt someone if I drive when I've been drinking.

MY PROS AND CONS FOR SUBSTANCE USE

PART I: IDENTIFYING THE PROS AND CONS

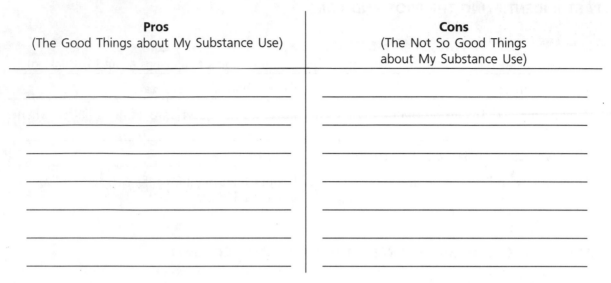

Pros	**Cons**
(The Good Things about My Substance Use)	(The Not So Good Things about My Substance Use)

PART II: ASSIGNING IMPORTANCE TO THE PROS AND CONS

How important is each of the above items to you in making a decision about your substance use? (Write a number rating on the line next to each item.) Use the following choices:

1 = Slightly important
2 = Moderately important
3 = Very important
4 = Extremely important

P/C/P SESSION 9

Relationships

CHANGE PROCESS OBJECTIVE: ENVIRONMENTAL REEVALUATION

RATIONALE

Environmental reevaluation involves recognizing the effect that a behavior has on one's environment. For substance abusers, this includes the effect their use may have had on their families, work, and social life. This session stimulates clients to begin to think about the relationships in their lives. As they do so, it may become more and more evident that their substance abuse has caused negative consequences not only for themselves but also for their relationships with others.

CONTENT OBJECTIVES

Clients recognize that behavior can affect other people.
Clients identify current and potential relationships.
Clients discuss how relationships have changed.
Clients think about whether relationships have changed as a result of substance use.

MATERIALS REQUIRED

Copies of the following for distribution to each group member:
"My Relationships" handout (P/C/P-9.1)
"My Relationships (Example)" handout (P/C/P-9.2)

SESSION SUMMARY

The facilitator explains that as humans, we have an innate need to interact with other humans. He or she then conducts an exercise to demonstrate how an action by one person results in a *re*-action by another. Clients list the current relationships in their lives, as well as those that they would like to form. The group breaks into pairs and discusses how these relationships have changed over time. The facilitator asks clients to think about whether relationships have changed as a result of their substance use.

IMPLEMENTATION

Clients may be unaware or unwilling to accept that their substance use affects other people in their lives. In this session, conduct an exercise to help clients identify the relationships that are present in their lives and determine how connected they feel to these relationships. Then, introduce the idea of examining each relationship and how it may have changed over time. Remember that this is not a coercive exercise—you are simply attempting to help clients understand that their actions can have repercussions for other people in their lives. Listen empathetically as clients discuss their relationships, asking open-ended questions and reflecting on clients' answers to encourage elaboration. Clients may be particularly vulnerable as they discuss the impact their use has had on others. Be sure to model for the group a supportive, caring style.

Steps 1 and 2: Open the Session and Introduce the Topic

Begin today's session by introducing the topic of relationships. Explain that because we are human, there is an inherent need in each of us to interact with other humans. What clients sometimes forget is that actions cause "*re*-actions" in other people. Demonstrate this by having one member of the group begin a sentence using *one* word. Have the next person add *one* word to the sentence, and so on, until the sentence is complete. Explain that each person's word depended on the one just spoken, and without *all* of the words, there would have been no sentence. (*Note.* This activity can be extended by having the clients "tell a story" by adding phrases together instead of simply single words.)

Step 3: Identify Relationships

Distribute the "My Relationships" handout (P/C/P-9.1). Have clients write a list of people with whom they have relationships at the top of the handout (initials instead of full names are fine). Give prompts to help clients think of the people with whom they interact, such as family members, friends, co-workers, neighbors, and so on. This list may even include substance-using friends or other people related to clients' substance use. Clients can also write the names or initials of people with whom they *would like* to form relationships on this list. The intention is for *the client* to identify who is most important at the current time. The goal of this exercise is for clients to evaluate the relationships in their lives and to examine how their substance use enters into those relationships.

When they have finished the list of people, distribute the "My Relationships (Example)" handout (P/C/P-9.2). Explain to clients that this sample demonstrates how to complete the rest of this exercise. Have the clients identify those people on the list most important in their lives. Ask clients to write the initials of those people in the circle closest to "Me." Then, have clients go to the next circle and write the next closest people, and so on. For people with whom they would like to form relationships, clients can write the initials on the edge of the largest circle. Explain how the example does this. Walk among the group, helping as needed.

Step 4: Discuss How Relationships Have Changed

Break the group into pairs and ask clients to discuss how these relationships may have changed over time. Explain that relationships change for many reasons, but one reason could be because of the way that people act when they are drinking or using other drugs. Have clients draw a square around the initials of people with whom the relationship could use some improvement. Walk among the pairs and probe to see which relationships may have been affected by their substance use, and whether this is the reason that some people have a square around their name.

Step 5: Close the Session

Bring the large group back together and discuss the exercise. Ask if anyone would be willing to show his or her circles to the group. If so, thank clients for sharing their personal relationships and assure them of the group's support. Affirm self-motivating statements, particularly those about concern and intent to change. Ask group members to pay attention to their relationships in the coming months and to change the placement of initials on the circles if the relationships change as time passes. Also encourage clients to reevaluate periodically which relationships could use improvement.

STEP-BY-STEP SESSION TASKS

Step 1: Open the session and check in with the group (approximately 10 minutes).

Step 2: Introduce the topic: Relationships (approximately 10 minutes).

- Explain that humans have an innate need to interact with other humans.
- Demonstrate how behaviors between people are connected. Do this by having a client begin a sentence by saying *one* word.
- Have the client sitting next to him or her add *one* word, and so on, until the sentence is complete.

Step 3: Identify relationships (approximately 15 minutes).

- Distribute the "My Relationships" handout (P/C/P-9.1).

- Have clients write a list of people with whom they have relationships. These can be close relationships or acquaintances.
- Distribute the "My Relationships (Example)" handout (P/C/P-9.2).
- Give prompts to help clients think of the people with whom they interact.
- Clients can also write the names or initials of people with whom they *would like* to form relationships.
- Have clients begin with the circle closest to "Me" and write initials of the people that are the most important in their lives.
- Have clients move out to the next circle and write the next-closest people, and so on.
- For people with whom they would like to form relationships, clients can write the initials on the edge of the largest circle.
- Walk among the group, helping as needed.

Step 4: Discuss how relationships have changed (approximately 10 minutes).

- Divide the group into pairs.
- Have pairs discuss how these relationships may have changed over time.
- Ask clients to draw a square around names of people with whom the relationship could be improved.
- Explain that there are many reasons why relationships change, and that substance use is one of them.
- Walk among the pairs, inquiring as to whether substance use affected the relationships that need improvement.

Step 5: Close the session (approximately 10 minutes).

- Discuss the activity.
- Check in with the group.
- Ask clients to reevaluate their relationships in the coming months.

MY RELATIONSHIPS

Here are the names or initials of people with whom I have relationships, and some with whom I would like to form relationships:

How important are these above people to you? Write the names or initials of the people who are the most important to you in the circle marked "Me." Then, write the initials/names of the people to whom you feel the next closest, and so on.

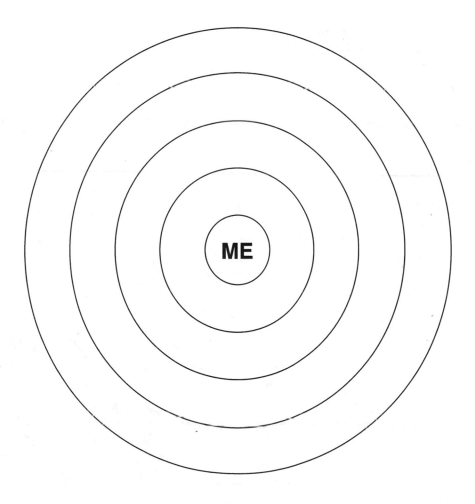

MY RELATIONSHIPS (EXAMPLE)

Here are the names or initials of people with whom I have relationships, and some with whom I would like to form relationships:

Bobby T.   Mom
Ryan R.   Dad
Lisa P.   Uncle Bill
Tyler D.   Jeremy L.

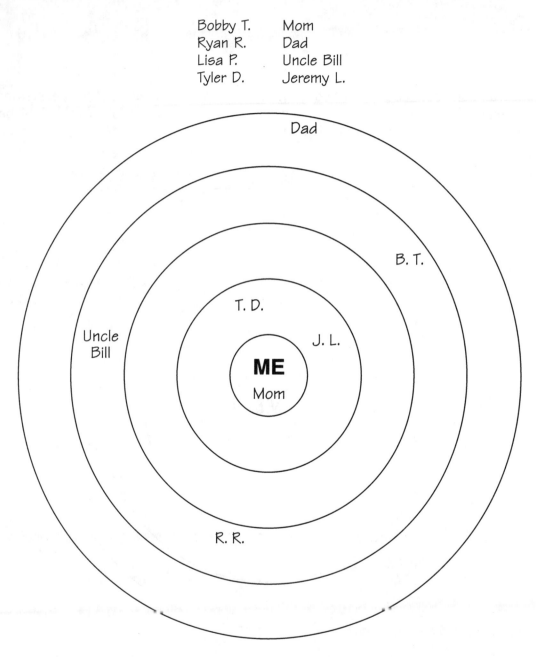

Roles

CHANGE PROCESS OBJECTIVE: ENVIRONMENTAL REEVALUATION

RATIONALE

Environmental reevaluation involves recognizing the effect that behavior has on one's life and environment. By identifying the roles that they fill, and how substance use has affected those roles, clients begin to recognize the effect that their alcohol or drug use has had on their lives.

CONTENT OBJECTIVES

Clients identify roles they hold.
Clients recognize how substance use has affected those roles.

MATERIALS REQUIRED

Copies of the "What Hats Do I Wear?" handout (P/C/P-10.1) for distribution to each group member.
Chalkboard/flipchart.

SESSION SUMMARY

The facilitator explains the concept of roles and assists the clients in identifying the roles that they currently play. Clients discuss how their substance use may have affected their roles.

IMPLEMENTATION

In the previous session, group members discussed how substance use might have affected their relationships with other people. While relationships involve roles (such as the caregiver role a parent plays to a child), there are also other roles in life through which we define ourselves (such as worker or student, or member of a softball team). Each role comes with particular requirements or expectations. In this session, assist clients in understanding that substance use may affect their ability to function in their *roles*. Clients will complete an exercise to clarify the roles that they play and then discuss how their drinking or drug use may have caused them difficulty in functioning in those roles.

(*Note.* This session differs from the previous one in that the focus is on how substance abuse has affected clients' ability to perform the functions that are expected in various areas of their lives rather than strictly on the relationships. This time, the discussion is not limited just to people in the clients' environment but includes other aspects of their environment that help them to define themselves.)

Steps 1 and 2: Open the Session and Introduce the Topic

Begin today's session with a discussion of roles. Using the previous descriptions, help clients understand what is meant by the term "role." Ask if the group has ever heard the phrase "He wears many different hats"? Explain that this means one person can function in several different *roles* even in a single day.

Step 3: Identify Personal Roles

Have the group generate a list of roles that people can fill and write this on the chalkboard/flipchart (e.g., student, son, daughter, friend, employee, etc.). Encourage clients to be creative and come up with a number or roles. It might help clients identify roles to have them think about situations in which people depend on them. Another way to do this is to define their roles in various relationships, then think about what are they expected to *do* in that relationship. The tasks or responsibilities that come with those relationships often determine that role.

Distribute the "What Hats Do I Wear?" handout (P/C/P-10.1). Have clients choose roles from those listed on the chalkboard/flipchart and decide which ones that they "fill" in their lives. Have them write the roles that they personally fill on the blank lines underneath the pictures of the hats. Emphasize that the roles do not have to correspond to the pictures of the hats. Walk among the clients during this exercise, helping them to generate appropriate roles as needed.

Step 4: Discuss How Substance Use Can Affect Roles

Explain to clients that each of the roles listed on the chalkboard/flipchart could be affected by substance use. If we do not meet expectations or responsibilities that are associated with our roles, certain consequences vary, depending on the role. For instance, in a client's role as an "employee," drinking alcohol may have caused significant problems in terms of career due to repeated terminations or a lack of good references. Choose two or three roles from the chalkboard/flipchart and point out how substance use could affect those roles. Facilitate a discussion regarding the roles that clients have identified on their handouts. Have clients think about how their drinking or drug use may hindered their ability to function in that role. Ask clients whether substance use has caused any previous roles to come to an end, or how it could prevent them from starting new roles in the future. Summarize periodically and reflect clients' expressions of concern and statements of intention to change.

Step 5: Close the Session

Briefly check in with the group and summarize today's session. Tell the group that it can be interesting to see how roles can change as time passes. Encourage clients to re-evaluate periodically the roles that they fill and how their personal behaviors are affecting those roles.

STEP-BY-STEP SESSION TASKS

Step 1: Open the session and check in with the group (approximately 10 minutes).

Step 2: Introduce the topic: Roles (approximately 10 minutes).

- Help clients understand the term "role."
- Explain that people can function in numerous roles, even during a single day.
- Ask if the group has heard the phrase "He wears many hats."

Step 3: Identify personal roles (approximately 15 minutes).

- Have clients be as creative and thorough as possible in generating a list of roles that people can fill; write the list on a chalkboard/flipchart.
- Distribute the "What Hats Do I Wear?" handout (P/C/P-10.1).
- Have clients identify several of the roles that they fill using the list on the chalkboard/handout for suggestions.
- Tell clients to write these roles on the blank lines underneath each hat on the handout.
- Emphasize that *the role does not have to correspond to the pictures of the hats; these are just examples.*

Step 4: Discuss how substance use can influence roles (approximately 20 minutes).

- Remind clients that they have seen how substance use may have affected their relationships with others.

- Explain that each of the roles listed on the chalkboard/flipchart could be affected by substance use as well.
- Choose two or three roles from the chalkboard/flipchart as examples and point out how substance use could affect those roles.
- Facilitate a discussion about the roles that clients have identified on their handouts.
- Ask group members whether substance use has caused any previous roles to come to an end, or how it might prevent them from starting new roles in the future.

Step 5: Close the session (approximately 10 minutes).

- Briefly check in with the group.
- Summarize the session, focusing on clients' self-motivational statements, particularly expressions of concern and intention to change.
- Encourage clients to reevaluate periodically the roles that they fill and how their personal behaviors are affecting those roles.

WHAT HATS DO I WEAR?

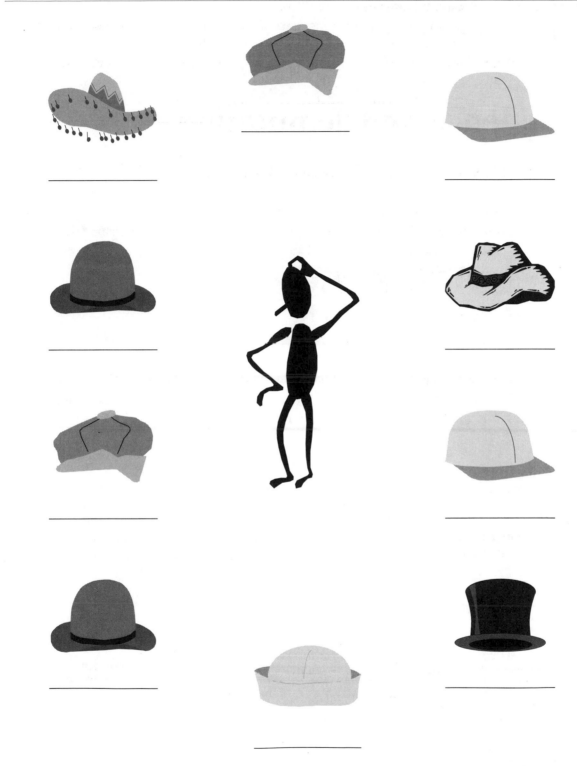

Confidence and Temptation

CHANGE PROCESS OBJECTIVE: SELF-EFFICACY

RATIONALE

Self-efficacy involves a person's confidence in knowing that he or she can take the steps necessary to accomplish a desired behavior. The focus of this session is on helping clients to identify the situations in which they are most tempted to use substances and to assess (and increase) their confidence to refrain from using in those same situations.

CONTENT OBJECTIVES

Clients identify situations in which they are most tempted to use substances.
Clients assess their confidence to refrain from use in tempting situations.
Clients discuss the implications of their varying levels of temptation and confidence.

MATERIALS REQUIRED

Copies of the following for distribution to each group member:
"The Most Tempting Times for Me Are . . . " handout (P/C/P-11.1)
"The Hardest Times for Me Are . . . " handout (P/C/P-11.2)

SESSION SUMMARY

Clients identify the situations in which they are most tempted to use substances and then assess their confidence to refrain from using in those same situations.

IMPLEMENTATION

In this session, clients first identify those times that are the most tempting (triggers) and then these times when they are the most confident that they will abstain. Next, they compare the two.

Steps 1 and 2: Open the Session and Introduce the Topic

Briefly check in with the group and introduce the topic by explaining the concepts of temptation and confidence. Tell clients that, today, they will assess their levels of temptation to use substances in certain "high-risk" situations, and their confidence that they could refrain from using in those same situations.

Step 3: Identify Triggers

Distribute the "The Most Tempting Times for Me Are . . . " handout (P/C/P-11.1). Tell clients that you will read each item aloud and ask them to make a check mark in the blanks beside each situation where they would be very tempted to use alcohol or other drugs. Tell them to mark as many situations as they need. When they have finished, they should total the checks for each column and write the totals on the lines at the bottom.

Step 4: Explain Trigger Categories

When clients have finished, explain that there are four areas in which people are most tempted to relapse: when they are experiencing negative emotional states, physical problems, or social pressure, and when they have the urge to drink (Marlatt & Gordon, 1985; DiClemente et al., 1995). Explain that each column on their handout represents one of these categories of trigger situations. Tell clients that the column in which they have placed the most checks is the category in which they are most tempted to drink or use drugs. Distribute "The Hardest Times for Me Are . . . " handout (P/C/P-11.2) and read the category descriptions while the group follows along. Facilitate a group discussion about clients' experience with the exercise. Did anyone learn anything surprising about their temptations to use?

Step 5: Identify Confident Situations

Tell clients that they are going to do one more thing with the "trigger description" handout, that while temptation is important, it is only part of the picture. Another very important piece of information is their confidence level in each situation. Explain that at the bottom of each column, there is a question that asks how *confident* they are that they would *not* use alcohol or drugs in that type of situation. At one end of the scale below the question are the words "Not at all confident" and at the other end, "Very confident." Ask clients to make a slash mark on the line that best represents, for each category, how confident they are that they would not use substances.

Step 6: Compare Temptation and Confidence

When clients have finished, ask them to look first at each column and think about their levels of temptation for that category, and then at their confidence rating for that same category. In some cases, a client will not be very tempted to use, and will have high confidence; in that case, this category is not of particular concern for that client. In other categories, clients may see that they are not only tempted but also confident. They do not have to be quite so concerned about this type of situation, but they may want to think about whether their confidence appraisal is realistic. Explain that sometimes people overestimate their confidence, which can lead to problems. Tell clients that they should be most concerned about situations in which they have high temptation levels but low confidence. It will be important for them to learn how to avoid these situations whenever possible, and to learn alternatives to using alcohol and drugs when these situations arise.

Step 7: Close the Session

Briefly check in with the group and summarize the session. Point out that both confidence and temptation often change as time passes. Encourage clients to continue to be aware of their temptation and confidence in various situations throughout the next few weeks. Suggest that they "revisit" this exercise periodically to monitor changes in their temptation and confidence.

STEP-BY-STEP SESSION TASKS

Step 1: Open the session and check in with the group (approximately 10 minutes).

Step 2: Introduce the topic: confidence and temptation (approximately 5 minutes).

- Explain that clients will assess their own areas of temptation to use substances and their confidence about being able to avoid using in tempting situations.

Step 3: Identify Triggers (approximately 10 minutes).

- Distribute the "Most Tempting Times for Me Are . . ." handout (P/C/P-11.1).
- Read each item aloud while clients make a check mark next to each situation where they would be very tempted to use alcohol or other drugs.
- Instruct clients to total the checks for each column and write the totals on the lines at the bottom.

Step 4: Explain trigger categories (approximately 10 minutes).

- Explain that there are four areas in which people are most tempted to use substances: when they are experiencing negative emotional states, physical problems, or social pressure, and when they have the urge to drink or use drugs.

- Tell clients those columns where they placed the most checks represent the areas in which they are most tempted to drink or use drugs.
- Distribute "The Hardest Times for Me Are . . ." handout (P/C/P-11.2) and read the category descriptions to the group.
- Facilitate a discussion about clients' experiences with the exercise. (What did they learn?)

Step 5: Identify confident situations (approximately 10 minutes).

- Explain that clients' level of confidence in each tempting situation is also very important.
- Point out that at the bottom of each column on the (same) handout there is a place to mark how *confident* they would be that they would not use in each situation.
- Ask clients to make a slash mark on the line that best represents, for each category, how confident they are that they would *not* use substances.

Step 6: Compare temptation and confidence (approximately 10 minutes).

- Ask clients to look at each column and think about their levels of temptation for that category and then at their confidence rating for that same category. Point out that they should be most concerned about categories where they are very tempted and not very confident. Also discuss the idea of "inflated" confidence.

Step 7: Close the session (approximately 5 minutes).

- Discuss the activity (approximately 10 minutes).
- Check in with the group.
- Ask clients to pay particular attention to areas where they are most tempted and least confident between now and the next session.

THE MOST TEMPTING TIMES FOR ME ARE . . .

Place a check mark in the blanks below for the situations in which you would be most tempted to use alcohol or drugs. (Mark as many situations as you need.) Then, add the checks for each column and write the total on the line.

_____ When I am having withdrawal symptoms.

_____ When I have the urge to try just one drink or drug.

_____ When I want to test my willpower.

_____ When I am feeling a physical need or craving.

_____ When I have an urge or impulse to take a drug or drink that catches me unprepared.

_____ When I have a headache.

_____ When I am concerned about someone.

_____ When I dream about using alcohol or drugs.

_____ When I am physically tired.

_____ When I'm experiencing some physical pain or injury.

_____ When I am feeling depressed.

_____ When I am very worried.

_____ When I feel like blowing up because of frustration.

_____ When I feel that everything is going wrong for me.

_____ When I am feeling angry inside.

_____ When I am on vacation and want to relax.

_____ When I am offered a drink or a drug in a social situation.

_____ When I see others drinking or using drugs at a bar or party.

_____ When people I used to drink or do drugs with encourage me to drink or use drugs.

_____ When I am excited or celebrating with others.

TOTAL: _____

THE HARDEST TIMES FOR ME ARE . . .

When I'm struggling with withdrawal

This category represents temptation to use when you are experiencing cravings and urges, or when you are having withdrawal symptoms.

Withdrawal symptoms include DT's (seeing things that really are not there), shakes, hot or cold flashes, vomiting, and so on. These things happen because the body has become used to having alcohol or drugs in its system, and is trying to "get used to" living without them.

How confident are you that you would not use alcohol or other drugs in this type of situation?

1   2   3   4   5
Not at all   Very
confident   confident

When I have physical and other troubles

This category represents temptation to use when you are not feeling well physically, or when you are in pain, such as when you have a headache or are physically tired.

This category also represents temptation to use when you are worried about someone or even when you "dream" about using alcohol or drugs.

How confident are you that you would not use alcohol or other drugs in this type of situation?

1   2   3   4   5
Not at all   Very
confident   confident

When I have negative feelings

This category represents temptation to use when you are upset emotionally, like when you feel sad or worried.

It also represents temptation to use when you are having a bad day and everything is going wrong for you, or when you are feeling frustrated and angry.

How confident are you that you would not use alcohol or other drugs in this type of situation?

1   2   3   4   5
Not at all   Very
confident   confident

When I am in social or positive situations

This category represents temptation to use during times when you are in social situations or just "hanging out" with your friends. Or when people with whom you used to use alcohol and drugs are drinking or high and want you to "join in."

It also represents times when you want to celebrate something good, or when you just want to relax and have fun.

How confident are you that you would not use alcohol or other drugs in this type of situation?

1   2   3   4   5
Not at all   Very
confident   confident

Problem Solving

CHANGE PROCESS OBJECTIVE: SELF-EFFICACY

RATIONALE

Self-efficacy involves a person's confidence in knowing that he or she can take the steps necessary to accomplish a desired behavior. Equipping clients with problem-solving skills helps them to think through situations and plan the steps to take rather than responding solely based on their emotions, feelings, or instincts. When clients experience success in problem solving, their self-efficacy is increased.

CONTENT OBJECTIVES

Clients learn to think through a problem.
Clients review an example of problem solving.

MATERIALS REQUIRED

Copies of the following for distribution to each group member:
    "Problem-Solving Examples" handout (P/C/P-12.1)
    "Choosing a Solution: 'Dave's Options' " handout (P/C/P-12.2)

SESSION SUMMARY

Facilitators teach clients how to solve problems by brainstorming options, listing and weighing the pros and cons, taking consequences into consideration, and then making a design based on this information. Clients review a detailed example of this process.

IMPLEMENTATION

Many people who abuse substances report that when they are in stressful situations, they tend to react based on their emotions rather than thinking through the situation and the possible consequences of their actions. The acquisition of problem-solving skills can help clients make decisions that are more reasoned. These skills are not only beneficial in helping clients avoid alcohol and drug use but also they can help in many other life situations. As clients generate problem-solving ideas in today's session, affirm them and express your confidence in their abilities to deal with stressful situations without using substances.

Steps 1 and 2: Open the Session and Introduce the Topic

Begin this session by checking in with the group. Then explain that when faced with difficult situations, people often respond based upon their emotions, feelings, or instincts, and how decisions based on emotion often do not take into consideration potential consequences and can lead to problematic situations. The benefit of learning problem-solving skills is that it can help people make better decisions by providing rational, logical thought process to follow before acting, rather than simply responding with impulsive behaviors. Discuss this and other benefits with the group. Remind clients of the decisional balancing exercises that they completed in a previous session. Note that in today's session you will talk about how to solve problems using a similar technique.

Step 3: Identify Options

Distribute the "Problem-Solving Examples" handout (P/C/P-12.1). Read the first example out loud, while the group follows along. Then, begin a discussion by writing "What can he do?" on a chalkboard/flipchart. Ask the group to come up with a list of options for the person in this situation. Write them on the board as group members respond. Prompt them with suggestions such as "What are different methods of transportation that Dave can use?" (i.e., take a taxi or a bus, ask a friend).

Explain that clients have just completed one step of the problem-solving process: "brainstorming." In brainstorming, clients write down as many ideas as they can think of, *without judging or eliminating options*. Writing down "crazy" or unrealistic ideas can be helpful because they might spark other, more realistic ideas. Brainstorming is often helpful in a group, or with another person, because sometimes ideas "pop up" when someone else mentions another idea.

Step 4: Choose the Best Solution

Introduce the next step in the problem-solving process: For each idea generated, list its positives and negatives, its pros and cons. These consequences can either be for yourself or for other people. Distribute the "Choosing a Solution: 'Dave's Options' " handout (P/C/P-12.2). Read across each row on the chart, clarifying points for clients as needed.

Explain that the "best" solution is found in the option with the most positive consequences. Point out that clients can eliminate options by counting the number of consequences that negatively affect themselves or others in their lives.

Step 5: Close the Session

Briefly check in with the group and summarize the session. Explain that the problem-solving process can be completed in advance for problems that have not yet occurred. For instance, you can think about a problem that you might be faced with and come up with solutions before it even occurs. Have the group think of a few situations where knowing the "answers" ahead of time would be helpful. Encourage clients to practice using problem-solving skills during the next few months.

STEP-BY-STEP SESSION TASKS

Step 1: Open the session and check in with the group (approximately 10 minutes).

Step 2: Introduce the topic: Problem solving.

Step 3: Identify options (approximately 10 minutes).

- Distribute the "Problem-Solving Examples" handout (P/C/P-12.1).
- Read the first example aloud.
- Have clients brainstorm options.

Step 4: Choose the best option (approximately 10 minutes).

- Remind clients how to list the pros and cons.
- Distribute the "Choosing a Solution: 'Dave's Options' " handout (P/C/P-12.2).
- Read the chart aloud and discuss with clients.
- Explain that the best option is the one with the most "pros" and *positive* consequences for yourself and others.
- Point out that options can be eliminated by counting the number of "cons" or consequences that negatively affect yourself or others.

Step 5: Close the session (approximately 10 minutes).

- Briefly check in with the group.
- Summarize the session.
- Affirm clients' problem-solving ideas.
- Express your confidence in clients' abilities to deal with stressful situations in positive ways.

PROBLEM-SOLVING EXAMPLES

EXAMPLE #1

Dave had a job interview on Tuesday morning. He was excited about the job prospect but was worried about how to get there, since he had no transportation. Dave was new to the city and had no money. He had borrowed a suit from a friend, so that he could make a good impression. This job was his only hope of paying his bills for the month. The interview was to be at 9:00 A.M. and he had to get all the way across town.

What could he do?

EXAMPLE #2

Mike had just moved to Pittsburgh and had been hired as a mail carrier. He liked the job well enough, but he kept getting into trouble with his supervisor. He was great at separating the envelopes and letters at the post office, but he could never finish his mail route on time. He kept forgetting which houses were where, and he almost always got lost. By the time he finished delivering that mail the following day, he would be behind on the next day's mail, and he always had trouble catching up. On Friday, his supervisor told him that he had better learn his route before Monday or he would be fired.

What can he do?

CHOOSING A SOLUTION: "DAVE'S OPTIONS"

Possible solution	Positive consequences (pros)	Negative consequences (cons)
Take the bus	1. Would save money	1. Bus could be late 2. Have to read the bus schedule 3. Will have to borrow money from a friend
Take a taxi	1. Quick 2. Cab driver can find the location	1. Very expensive 2. Have to chat with cab driver 3. Will have to borrow money from a friend
Get a ride from a friend	1. Might be free 2. Friend can encourage you on the way	1. Might have to chip in for gas money 2. Will owe friend a favor
Walk	1. Will get exercise	1. Might sweat on the way 2. Longest travel time

Setting a Goal and Preparing to Change

CHANGE PROCESS OBJECTIVE: SELF-LIBERATION

RATIONALE

Self-liberation involves making a commitment to behavior change. In this session, clients are asked to set a goal about their substance use and create a plan by which to meet that goal. In thinking about their goals and committing to a change plan, clients will be using the change process of self-liberation.

CONTENT OBJECTIVES

Clients learn about setting appropriate goals.
Clients create a goal statement and a change plan to meet that goal.

MATERIALS REQUIRED

Copies of the following for distribution to each group member:
  "Goal Setting and Change Plan (Example)" handout (P/C/P-13.1)
  "My Goal Setting and Change Plan" handout (P/C/P-13.2)

SESSION SUMMARY

The facilitator leads a discussion about goals. Clients identify times in the past when they have successfully set and met goals, and discuss the obstacles they faced while do-

113

ing so. Group members identify a goal about their substance use and create a plan that details the steps they will take to reach that goal.

IMPLEMENTATION

Helping clients set clear and realistic goals facilitates change. The development of a change plan can help solidify and assist clients in reaching their goals. In an earlier session, clients identified their values and ways in which their substance use conflicts with those values. This session is designed to help clients use that awareness to identify and clarify their goals, particularly those related to their substance use.

As clients move from the early stages into preparation, they typically become ready to set a goal with regard to their substance use. Oftentimes, a plan will have started to emerge during the earlier sessions, and they will have begun to think of ways to reach these goals. It can be helpful for clients to write out these plans and to identify people in their lives who can help them as they carry out their plan. It is also important for them to identify and anticipate possible barriers to reaching their goals. While these goal-setting and change plan exercises can be beneficial for clients in precontemplation and contemplation stages, they are most useful for those clients who are in the preparation stage. This session is an important "bridge" between the early stage sessions and the action–maintenance sessions.

(*Note*. By this time, most clients will be ready to set a goal and develop a plan to change their substance use, even if it is a reduction in the amount of substance use rather than abstinence. If clients express that they do not plan to change their use, they can either complete the change plan exercise with the goal of "staying the same" in terms of their use, or alternatively, they may choose a different behavior that they wish to change. The goal is to help clients learn how to develop a workable plan, anticipate potential barriers, and identify people in their environment who can assist them in their change attempts.)

Steps 1 and 2: Open the Session and Introduce the Topic

Remind clients of the session in which they discussed their values. During that session, they explored the areas in which their substance-using behavior was discrepant with their values. At this point, clients are likely to be ready to set goals related to their use. Goals should be well thought out and realistic. Explain that a realistic goal is attainable and one for which they can identify a plan by which it can be reached. For example, the goal "I will never again drink alcohol" is not realistic *unless* it is accompanied by a plan that the client will use to attain it (such as attending AA meetings, avoiding drinking buddies, and so on). By having a plan, clients are much more likely to prevail over obstacles and to be successful in their change attempts. Tell clients that today's session will lead them through this process.

Step 3: Discuss Goals

Facilitate a group discussion about goals. Begin by asking clients to discuss times in the past when they have set goals for themselves and been successful in meeting them. By remembering past successes, clients begin to feel more confident about their abilities to meet future goals. After clients have thought about goals they have reached, ask questions such as the following:

- "What steps did you take in attaining your goal?"
- "What obstacles did you face?"
- "How were you able to overcome those obstacles?"

Step 4: Create a Goal Statement and Change Plan

Distribute the "Goal Setting and Change Plan (Example)" handout (P/C/P-13.1). Read through the handout, describing how to complete the sections one at a time. The example change plan provided in the manual provides prompts for you to use when explaining each section.

Distribute the "My Goal Setting and Change Plan" handout (P/C/P-13.2). Ask clients to write the goal in the space at the top and think about a goal for their own substance use. They will need to be as specific as they can by recording the substance(s) they are referring to and the exact change they want to make. Some clients will want to quit using the substance(s) all together; others might opt to reduce their use.

Ask clients to be as realistic as they can in choosing their goals. Explain that they sometimes set goals that are too ambitious, so they set themselves up for failure. (Assure them that if this happens, it will most likely become evident in the process of developing their change plan, and at that point, they may modify their goal.) Other clients may set their goals too low and decide to revise them after going through the change plan process and the group discussion.

Once clients have identified their goals, ask if anyone is willing to share his or her goal aloud. With a few clients, demonstrate the completion of the rest of the form. Asking open-ended questions such as "How do you think you might do that?" and "What might get in the way?" can help clients develop their plans. Summarizing clients' goals and change plans aloud can be helpful in that it often helps clients strengthen their resolve and allows them to think about any weaknesses in their plan.

Have clients complete the rest of the worksheet, identifying people who might help them and any barriers that might get in their way. If clients ask for assistance, you may wish to offer some ideas or ask other group members for input. Your goal during this exercise, though, is to elicit ideas from clients, not to prescribe a plan for them.

Step 5: Close the Session

Congratulate clients on the very important step they have taken today. Tell them that the formation of a goal statement and change plan is critical in the process of change. Inform them that they may wish to revise their plan as they try new behaviors and learn more about the change that they are attempting to make. Affirm clients and remind them that you and the group are there to support them as they implement their plans.

STEP-BY-STEP SESSION TASKS

Step 1: Open the session and check in with the group (approximately 10 minutes).

Step 2: Introduce the topic: Setting a goal and preparing to change (approximately 10 minutes).

Step 3: Discuss goals (approximately 10 minutes).

- Facilitate a group discussion about goals.
- Ask clients to discuss times in the past when they have set goals for themselves and have been successful in meeting those goals.
- Discuss this further by using prompts about what obstacles the clients faced in meeting goals and the steps they took to achieve the goal (approximately 20 minutes).

Step 4: Create a goal statement and change plan.

- Distribute the "Goal Setting and Change Plan (Example)" (P/C/P-13.1) and "My Goal Setting and Change Plan" (P/C/P-13.2) handouts.
- Ask clients to think about a goal for substance use and write this at the top of the page.
- Have clients be as realistic as they can and set goals that are very meaningful for them.
- Ask if anyone is willing to share his or her goal aloud.
- Demonstrate the completion of the rest of the form few client.
- Summarize this client's goal and change plans aloud.
- Have clients complete the rest of the worksheet.

Step 5: Close the session (approximately 10 minutes).

- Briefly check in with clients.
- Summarize the session.
- Affirm clients for their progress.
- Express your confidence in each client's ability to accomplish his or her goals.
- Tell clients that they may wish to revise their plan as they try new behaviors and learn more about the change that they are attempting to make.

GOAL SETTING AND CHANGE PLAN (EXAMPLE)

My problem substances are:

This includes a list of the substances that cause you problems.

My goal for changing my substance use is:

This includes the exact changes you plan to make. For example, if abstinence is not your immediate goal, by how much will you reduce your use? Be specific about amounts and plans. Here are two examples from other clients:

> *"My problem substances are alcohol and cocaine. I plan to quit using both of these substances and to remain abstinent."*

> *"My problem substances are alcohol and marijuana. I plan to reduce my alcohol use so that I drink only three drinks a day on the weekend and do not drink during the week. I do not plan to change my marijuana use."*

What steps I plan to take:

Be as specific as possible about the actions you will take to reach your goal. For example:

> *"I will stay away from my friends who use and I will avoid bars."*

> *"I will plan healthy activities, such as exercising, to combat boredom and help me cope with urges to use."*

What can get in the way:

Think about any barriers you might encounter as you work toward your goal. For example:

> *"I might get lonely or bored and want to spend time with old friends."*

> *"My cousin might try to talk me into using because he thinks that's how we can have a good time."*

People who can help me:

List people (or groups of people) who can help you as you work toward your goal. For example:

> *Other group members*
> *AA friends*
> *Larry and Sue*

MY GOAL SETTING AND CHANGE PLAN

My problem substances are:

My goal for changing my substance use is:

What steps I plan to take:

What can get in the way:

People who can help me:

Review and Termination

RATIONALE

In this session, clients think back over the course of the group meetings and discuss the progress they have made toward behavior change.

CONTENT OBJECTIVES

Clients review the topics covered during the course of the group.
Clients discuss changes and progress group members have made.
Clients engage in termination activities.

MATERIALS REQUIRED

In advance of the session, prepare note cards that list several accomplishments or successes made by each client in the course of the group.
Copics of the "Review" handout (P/C/P-14.1) for distribution to each group member
Chalkboard/flipchart

SESSION SUMMARY

As facilitator, review all of the topics and techniques covered during the course of the group. Also, assist with termination by leading a discussion of how the group has affected clients, what they expect in the coming weeks without the group, and "where they can go from here." Share a few accomplishments/successes for each group member; then give clients note cards to take with them, on which these accomplishments/successes are written.

IMPLEMENTATION

Many people have difficulty in ending relationships in a healthy way, and a therapeutic setting provides an opportunity to practice this skill. In today's session, help group members do this by summarizing their experiences during the group. Also, review each of the topics covered during the group.

Steps 1 and 2: Open the Session and Introduce the Topic

Begin by briefly checking in with the group; then, introduce the topic by explaining that, since this is the final session, you will review all of the topics covered throughout the course of the group. Point out that you will be helping clients to summarize their experiences during the group.

Step 3: Review the Group Topics

Explain that because you have covered so much information over the last several sessions, you will review the topics. Distribute the "Review" handout (P/C/P-14.1). Read several of the topics and their respective questions aloud, discussing them with clients. Ask clients how their answers differ now from when you first discussed the subject.

Step 4: Conduct a Staging Exercise

Ask clients to think about whether they feel they have moved forward or stayed "about the same" in terms of their alcohol/drug use, answering only to themselves. On a chalkboard/flipchart draw the stages of change diagram (see Session 1) and briefly summarize each stage. Ask clients to look at each stage as you describe their current stage. Have clients think about whether their stage is different now than it was earlier in the group, answering only to themselves.

Step 5: Facilitate Termination Process

Point out that this group has most likely been a source of support to its members for quite some time, and clients should not feel "abandoned" simply because they will no longer meet as a group on a regular basis. Remind clients that they have other sources of support available to them in their lives, and perhaps now some of the other group members would be considered supporters, too. [This would be an appropriate place to provide the telephone number of a local crisis hotline or to review clients' options in the event of a substance-use emergency (such as contacting your staff if appropriate, going to the emergency room at a local hospital, and so on).]

Explain that a helpful way to close a treatment group is to think back over the course of the group and see how it has affected your life. Facilitate a group discussion about this particular group using several of the following prompts, one question at a time; model appropriate termination skills by being the first one to answer; then, open each question up for group discussion:

- "Name two things you have learned in the group."
- "How has the group affected your life?"
- "Name one positive thing about at least one other group member."
- "What will be different for you without the group?"
- "Where do you think you will 'go from here'?"
- "Anything else you would like to say?"

Some of the clients in this group may move on to the action–maintenance group detailed in the second half of this manual. Others may go out on their own. For these clients, it would be helpful to suggest places they can go for support as they move toward taking action, such as AA or other self-help groups.

Step 6: Close the Session

Summarize the session, then read the "brief summary" note cards you have prepared for each client (see "Materials Required" for further information). For example, "Bob, you have become more comfortable in talking about your substance use during this group. I can tell you have done a lot of thinking about your situation" or "Marilyn, you have a lot of insight and have helped other group members see their positive qualities." Give the note card to each client after you read it, so he or she can take this home as a reminder of his or her progress. If you feel that it is appropriate, you can encourage the other group members to clap or otherwise congratulate each other as you read the cards. Check in with the clients one last time to close the group.

STEP-BY-STEP SESSION TASKS

Step 1: Open the session and check in with the group (approximately 5 minutes).

Step 2: Introduce the topic: Review and termination (approximately 5 minutes).

- Explain that because this is the final group, you will review all of the topic covered along the course of the group.
- Point out that you will be helping clients to summarize their experiences during the group (i.e., help with termination).

Step 3: Review the group topics (approximately 15 minutes).

- Distribute the "Review" handout (P/C/P-14.1).
- Read several of the topics and their respective questions aloud.
- Discuss these with the clients.
- Ask clients how their answers differ now from when you first discussed the subject.

Step 4: Conduct a staging exercise (approximately 10 minutes).

- Ask the clients to think about whether they have moved forward, backward, or stayed "about the same" regarding their alcohol/drug use during the group; have them answer only to themselves.
- Draw the stages of change diagram on a chalkboard/flipchart.
- Summarize each of the stages, having clients decide what stage they are currently in as you describe them.
- Discuss this activity with the group.

Step 5: Facilitate termination process (approximately 15 minutes).

- Point out that the clients have all identified supporters in their lives, and some of the group members may have been added to that list.
- Emphasize that clients should not feel abandoned with the close of the group, since they still have their supporters.
- Provide a local crisis hotline telephone number or explain the options clients have in the event of an emergency.
- Facilitate a discussion regarding how clients feel that the group has affected their lives (be the first one to do this, using the prompts).

Step 6: Close the session (approximately 10 minutes).

- Summarize the session.
- Affirm each client for the progress he or she has made.
- Read each of the note cards that you have prepared (see "Materials Required").
- Give the note card to each member after you read it so he or she can take it as a reminder of his or her progress.
- Check in with the group.

REVIEW

Listed below are the topics we have covered along the course of this group. Each topic has one or two questions to help you remember specific information and to see if your answers are different now from when the group began.

- The Stages of Change—What are the five stages? What stage are you in?

- A Day in the Life—How much and how often are you using?

- Physiological Effects of Alcohol and Drugs—How can alcohol and other drugs affect your body?

- Expectations—What do you expect with regard to drinking alcohol or using drugs? Are these expectations realistic?

- Expressions of Concern—Who is concerned about your substance use?

- Values—Does your substance use agree with your values or not?

- Pros and Cons—What are the positives and negatives of substance use? How do these "weigh" against each other?

- Relationships—Does your substance use affect your relationships with others?

- Roles—Does your substance use affect the roles that you play in life?

- Confidence and Temptation—When are you tempted to use substances, and when are you confident that you will not?

- Problem Solving—What are the steps to problem solving?

- Setting a Goal and Preparing to Change—What is your goal? What are the barriers to this goal?

PART III

Making Changes in Substance Use

A/M Sequence: Action–Maintenance

CLIENT HANDOUTS

A/M-1.1. Stages of Change, 133

A/M-1.2. Where Am I?, 134

A/M-2.1. When Am I the Most Tempted to Use?, 139

A/M-3.1. Meditation, 145

A/M-4.1. Rewarding My Successes, 150

A/M-5.1. Effective Communication, 155

A/M-6.1. Practicing Refusals, 160

A/M-7.1. Managing Criticism, 165

A/M-8.1. Maladaptive Thoughts, 171

A/M-9.1. To Manage Cravings and Urges I Can . . . , 176

A/M-10.1. Alternatives to Using, 181

A/M-11.1. Review, 186

A/M-11.2. My Action Plan, 188

A/M-12.1. What Can I Do after a Slip?, 193

A/M-13.1. Where Do I Get Help?, 198

A/M-14.1. Needs Assessment, 203

A/M-14.2. Resource Guide, 204

A/M-15.l. Review, 210

The Stages of Change

CHANGE PROCESS OBJECTIVE: CONSCIOUSNESS RAISING

RATIONALE

The stages of change offer an integrative framework for understanding and facilitating behavior change. The goal of the first session in this second sequence is to help clients understand the stages of change model, and to explain that the approach to be used by all group members is one of nonconfrontation, empathy, and respect. It can serve as a refresher for clients who have gone through the first group sequence of it may be skipped if the two sequences are run together as one continuous sequence.

CONTENT OBJECTIVES:

Learn stages of change model.
Complete staging exercise to determine own stage of change.

MATERIALS REQUIRED

Chalkboard/flipchart
Chalk or markers
Copies of the following for distribution to each group member:
　　"Stages of Change" handout (A/M-1.1)
　　"Where Am I?" handout (A/M-1.2)

SESSION SUMMARY

The facilitators introduces the concept of a motivational approach to behavior change. The approach to be taken by all members of the group should be one of empathy, acceptance, and respect for individual differences. Unlike some models of substance abuse treatment, this approach explicitly avoids confrontation. During this session, the group rules are established and the stages of change model is discussed. The facilitator reads vignettes for each of the stages aloud, having the clients choose which stage applies to each scenario. The clients complete a simple self-staging exercise.

IMPLEMENTATION

Explain to clients that you will be using a "motivational approach" in the group, which is quite different than any treatment experiences they may have had in the past. In introducing these motivational concepts to the group, you will be teaching them how to use this style in their interactions with one another. Since this group is very different from others in which they may have participated, it might take a while for them to get used to the style of interaction, and they may need gentle reminders as you progress through the early sessions. As you model this approach, group members will catch on. The "housekeeping" is also taken care of in this session (introductions, establishing the group rules, and so on).

Steps 1 and 2: Open the Session and Establish Group Rules

Begin this session by introducing yourself. Then have group members each introduce themselves and tell one thing they hope to get out of the group. Introduce the concept of a motivational approach to behavior change, telling clients that while you are the group "facilitator," each client also plays an important role in helping other group members as you go through this process together. Tell clients that you are here to help them learn more about themselves and decide whether there are any changes they would like to make. Assure them that while you have the knowledge and the skills to help them, ultimately, *if there is any changing to be done, they will be the ones to do it.* The responsibility for change is up to them, and you will not coerce them or try to force them to change in any way. Explain that this is also the approach you would like for clients to take toward one another: "In this group, we will avoid confrontation and, rather, help facilitate change in one another through supportive interactions." Thus, the approach to be taken by all members of the group should be one of empathy, acceptance, and respect for individual differences. *Emphasize that unlike some models of substance abuse treatment, this approach explicitly avoids confrontation.*

Since this is likely to be a new approach to most clients, spend a few minutes discussing how this approach feels to them. You may wish to tell them that research shows that a supportive, empathetic approach to behavior change is much more effective than a confrontational one.

Assist the group in developing its own rules, making sure to include the following:

- Respect self and others in the group.
- Refrain from interrupting or talking when others are talking.
- Avoid self "put-downs" or name calling.
- Be willing to give positive and negative feedback to others in respectful ways.
- Be willing to accept feedback from others without becoming verbally or physically aggressive/defensive.
- Maintain confidentiality outside of the group.

Step 3: Introduce Clients to the Stages of Change

Distribute the "Stages of Change" handout (A/M-1.1). Then, draw a stage diagram on a chalkboard/flipchart and introduce the clients to the stages:

- Precontemplation. The *precontemplation* stage is one in which individuals are either unconvinced that they have a problem or are unwilling to consider change.
- Contemplation. The *contemplation* stage is one in which a person is actively considering the possibility of change. People in this stage are evaluating options, but are not ready to take action at present.
- Preparation. In the *preparation* stage, individuals make a commitment as well as initial plans to change the behavior.
- Action. Once individuals take effective action to make the change, they are considered to be in the *action* stage. In action, a person adopts strategies to prevent a relapse and a return to the problem behavior.
- Maintenance. The *maintenance* stage of change is one in which the individual consolidates the change and integrates it into his or her lifestyle.

Explain that everyone goes through these stages as they are attempting to change behavior. However, it is also natural for people to "recycle" through (i.e., revisit) earlier stages several times before successfully making and maintaining the change. Explain that rather than being viewed as a failure, a "slip" can be seen as an opportunity to provide useful information and experiences for the next attempt.

Step 4: Conduct a Staging Exercise

Read the following vignettes aloud one at a time. After each scenario, ask group members which stage of change they think applies. Give "hints" as needed and refer to the staging diagram on the chalkboard/flipchart. Remind the clients that they can refer to their "Stages of Change" handout (A/M-1.1) as well.

Staging Vignettes

Joseph has been thinking about losing weight, but he just hasn't been able to start exercising like he used to. He has done sit-ups a few mornings during the last several weeks, and he has pumped up the tires on his bicycle. He has also talked to some of his friends who lift weights to see what their routines are. After lunch today, though, he took a nap instead of working out like he had planned. [Preparation]

Jane gets tired of everyone nagging at her to stop smoking. "Why don't they just leave me alone?" she says. It's bad enough that they raised the price of cigarettes this year, and now she can't even smoke in her office during the day. While she's outside on her break she thinks, "I can't get any work done without a cigarette. How do they expect me to finish this project on time if I have to keep coming outside to think?" [Precontemplation]

Marcus is proud of himself. He has gone for 2 weeks without taking a drink. He has started "hanging out" with some new friends at work who don't drink either, and his work has improved; his boss even noticed a difference! When he threw out all the alcohol from his house a few weeks ago, he wasn't sure if his resolve would last. Even though he's tempted to stop by the bar during "happy hour" after work, he has instead jogged in the park every evening since quitting. [Action]

Maria wonders if all this stuff about how caffeine can hurt your baby is true. She has been drinking five cups of coffee a day for as long as she can remember, and it hasn't seemed to do anything to her before. Still, she hasn't been able to sleep since she became pregnant, and now her stomach gets upset after even one cup of coffee. She saw some babies at the hospital that were really tiny, and the doctor says it's due to caffeine. "Maybe I should consider cutting down a little," she thinks. [Contemplation]

It's hard for Paul to believe it's been over 2 years since he used cocaine. The kids at the shelter where he volunteers remind him of himself at that age—it doesn't seem like so long ago he was addicted to crack himself. It hasn't been easy to stay clean, but it sure has been worth it. He recently told someone that it's nice to go to sleep at night without hating himself and everyone else. [Maintenance]

Step 5: Determine Clients' Stages of Change

Distribute the "Where Am I?" handout (A/M-1.2). Demonstrate how to determine stage using the cues on the handout. We suggest that you choose a nonthreatening behavior such as diet or exercise to use as an example. Next, instruct clients to think about their primary substance of abuse; have them read the cues and decide which stage they are in for that substance. Assist clients as needed. Facilitate a group discussion regarding clients' reactions to this exercise. Point out that the majority of the group is currently in the action and maintenance stages. Explain that this group has been designed specifically for clients who have begun to make changes in their substance use, and that it will help them to learn skills that will help them to continue making changes.

Step 6: Close the Session

Check in with group members to see if anyone has additional issues they want to discuss before the session ends. At the close of each session, summarize what has occurred in the group that day. Ask clients if you have missed anything or if they would like to add anything to your summary. Stress that this group is intended to help group members move through stages of change and that the facilitators will be available to assist in helping to deal with drug or alcohol problems. However, the decision of whether to change is up to each individual. No one will "force" them to do anything; the responsibility for change is theirs.

STEP-BY-STEP SESSION TASKS

Step 1: Open the session (approximately 10 minutes).

- Briefly introduce yourself to the group.
- Have group members introduce themselves and tell one thing they would like to get out of the group.

Step 2: Establish group rules (approximately 10 minutes).

- Facilitate discussion about the motivational approach.
- Assist clients in developing group rules.

Step 3: Introduce clients to the stages of change (approximately 15 minutes).

- Distribute the "Stages of Change" handout (A/M-1.1).
- Draw a stage diagram on a chalkboard/flipchart.
- Emphasize that people cycle through the stages and that a "slip" does not mean failure.

Step 4: Conduct a staging exercise (approximately 10 minutes).

- Read vignettes aloud one at a time (see "Implementation").
- Have clients guess which stage of change applies to each vignette after it is read.
- Refer to the staging diagram on the chalkboard/flipchart as you discuss each scenario.

Step 5: Determine clients' stages of change (approximately 20 minutes).

- Distribute the "Where Am I?" handout (A/M-1.2).
- Demonstrate how to determine stage, using an example of a nonthreatening problem behavior.

- Assist group members in determining their own stages of change.
- Facilitate a group discussion about this activity.

Step 6: Close the session (approximately 10 minutes).

- Summarize the session.
- Affirm clients for their participation.
- Check in with group members.

STAGES OF CHANGE

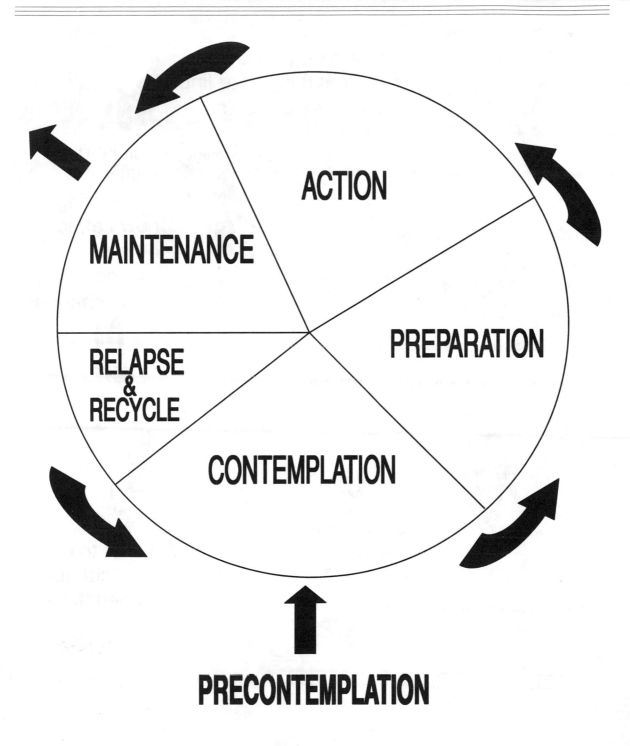

WHERE AM I?

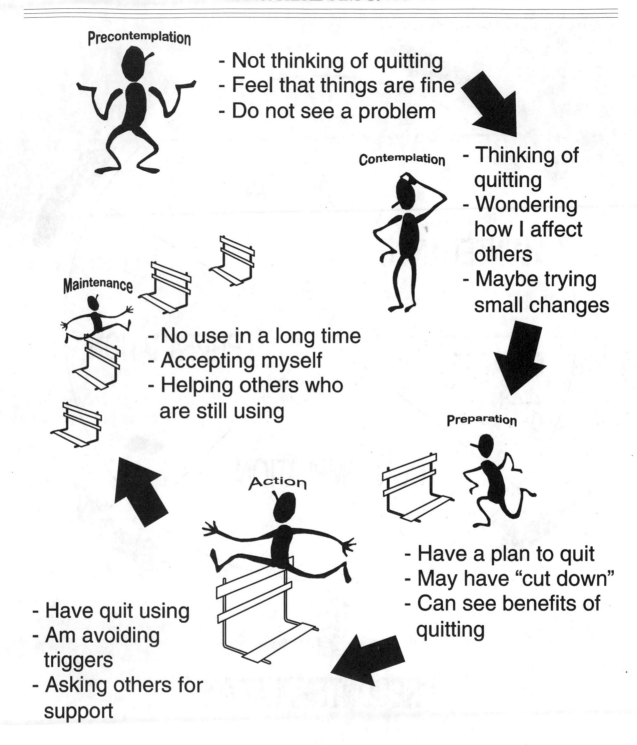

Precontemplation
- Not thinking of quitting
- Feel that things are fine
- Do not see a problem

Contemplation
- Thinking of quitting
- Wondering how I affect others
- Maybe trying small changes

Preparation
- Have a plan to quit
- May have "cut down"
- Can see benefits of quitting

Action
- Have quit using
- Am avoiding triggers
- Asking others for support

Maintenance
- No use in a long time
- Accepting myself
- Helping others who are still using

A/M SESSION 2

Identifying "Triggers"

CHANGE PROCESS OBJECTIVE: STIMULUS CONTROL

RATIONALE

Stimulus control involves avoiding or altering triggers for substance use so that the likelihood of using is lessened. This session begins to show clients how to use this change process to avoid substance use. It also assists clients in identifying their own specific triggers and helps them generate plans for avoiding or altering those triggers.

CONTENT OBJECTIVES

Clients identify situations or emotions that "trigger" alcohol or drug use.
Clients generate appropriate ways to avoid or alter those trigger situations.

MATERIALS REQUIRED

Copies of the "When Am I the Most Tempted to Use?" handout (A/M-2.1) for distribution to each group member

SESSION SUMMARY

Facilitators hold a discussion on the concept of "triggers." The clients complete an exercise in which they determine their own triggers. Group members discuss ways that they can successfully avoid or alter these trigger situations.

IMPLEMENTATION

It is often helpful for clients to identify the situations in which they are most tempted (and thereby most likely) to use alcohol or drugs. These high-risk situations usually trigger their impulse to drink or use drugs, and if they have not prepared in advance, their temptations may prove too strong to overcome. In this session, help clients to identify the "triggers" that tempt them to use, then help them generate ideas for altering or avoiding those cues. Ask open-ended questions and affirm clients as they identify triggers and options to use. Listen for statements about intention to change and reflect these, in particular, to the group.

Steps 1 and 2: Open the Session and Introduce the Topic

After briefly checking in with the group and reviewing the stages of change, introduce the concept of "triggers." Explain to clients that research shows that when faced with high-risk situations such as anger, anxiety, or social pressure to drink, people may either successfully perform adaptive coping behaviors or fail to cope. It is in these tempting situations that people are most likely to relapse (Marlatt & Gordon, 1985). Explain to clients that while these have been identified as the most common relapse determinants, not everyone has the same triggers. It is important for clients to develop coping skills that will help them overcome temptation in those areas where their triggers to use are the strongest. To facilitate this discussion, have the members think about the times when they have been the most tempted to use alcohol or drugs. Ask the group for examples of those times.

Step 3: Complete Exercise to Determine Triggers

Distribute the "When Am I the Most Tempted to Use?" handout (A/M-2.1). Read the directions and then the categories aloud, giving examples of the types of situations that fall under each. Have clients circle the category in which they would be most tempted to use alcohol or drugs. Tell clients about the extra space at the end of each category, which they can use to write specific examples.

Step 4: Discuss Ways to Avoid or Alter Trigger Situations

Explain that it is helpful to avoid or alter these trigger situations to keep from using alcohol or other drugs. Give examples of ways to do this such as the following:

1. Removing things from their homes that remind them of drinking or drug use.
2. Leaving places where other people are encouraging alcohol or other drug use.
3. Putting things around their homes or workplace that remind them not to engage in alcohol or drug use.
4. Relating less often to people who contribute to their alcohol/other drug use.

Facilitate a group discussion, asking clients to think about ways that they can avoid or alter their trigger situations. During the discussion, have clients write down suggestions for the category that is personally the most tempting. The following questions might prompt discussion that includes all four categories:

- "If you are tempted when you are in physical pain, what are options to avoid or alter those situations?"
- "If you are tempted when you are experiencing negative emotions, what options do you have to alter or avoid the situation?"
- "If social or positive situations tempt you the most, what things could you do to alter or avoid these situations?"
- "If you are tempted by cravings or urges, what could you do to alter these situations when they occur?"

Step 5: Close the Session

Briefly check in with the group members and summarize the session. Ask if you "got it all" or if you have left anything out. Explain that as the clients begin working on avoiding substance use, it will be very important to remember their own "triggers," so they can more effectively avoid using. Affirm clients for their participation.

STEP-BY-STEP SESSION TASKS

Step 1: Open the session (approximately 10 minutes).

- Check in with group members.
- Briefly review the stages of change.

Step 2: Introduce the session topic: Identifying triggers (approximately 15 minutes).

- Discuss the concept of "triggers" to use.
- Have group members give examples of situations in which they are the most tempted to use drugs or alcohol.

Step 3: Complete exercise to determine triggers (approximately 10 minutes).

- Distribute the "When Am I the Most Tempted to Use?" handout (A/M-2.1).
- Read the instructions and categories aloud, giving examples of each.
- Ask clients to circle the category that best describes when they are most tempted.
- Have clients write specific situations in the blank space following the category that tempts them most.

Step 4: Discuss ways to avoid or alter trigger situations (approximately 15 minutes).

- Give examples of ways to avoid or alter trigger situations.
- Facilitate a group discussion about ways to do this.
- During the discussion, have clients write down suggestions for the category that is personally the most tempting.

Step 5: Close the session (approximately 10 minutes).

- Summarize the session.
- Check in with group members.

WHEN AM I THE MOST TEMPTED TO USE?

It can be helpful to identify the times when you are really tempted to use alcohol or other drugs. By recognizing these "trigger" situations ahead of time, you have more of a chance to avoid or alter them when they occur. Circle the name of the category that best completes this sentence:

I am the most tempted to use during times of _____:

Negative Emotions:
Examples include:
- Anger
- Depression

Some Ways to Avoid or Alter This

Physical Pain:
Examples include:
- Aches and pains
- Tiredness

Some Ways to Avoid or Alter This

Social or Positive Events:
Examples include:
- Parties
- When happy or excited

Some Ways to Avoid or Alter This

Withdrawal:
- Cravings and urges
- Withdrawal symptoms

Some Ways to Avoid or Alter This

Managing Stress

CHANGE PROCESS OBJECTIVE: COUNTERCONDITIONING

RATIONALE

In a situation where it is difficult for clients to alter or avoid tempting cues, an effective strategy is to alter their *responses* to the cues. This change process of *counterconditioning* involves substituting healthy behaviors for unhealthy ones.

This session begins to show clients how to use counterconditioning to avoid substance use. The group is designed to teach clients how to replace habitual, unhealthy behaviors with appropriate, healthy ones, through the use of relaxation techniques.

CONTENT OBJECTIVES

Clients recognize how being in stressful situations can affect the body and behavior. Clients learn techniques to counter stress that might trigger use of alcohol or drugs. Clients practice relaxation techniques.

MATERIALS REQUIRED

Copies of the "Meditation" homework handout (A/M-3.1) for distribution to each group member

SESSION SUMMARY

Clients discuss examples of times when being in stressful situations affected their behavior. The facilitator explains the concept of relaxation (i.e., stress management).

Lead the group through two different relaxation exercises and distribute the handout on meditation for clients to take home.

IMPLEMENTATION

In today's session, you will be helping clients look more closely at stress, discussing which types of situations elicit physical and psychological signs of stress, and practicing relaxation techniques.

Steps 1 and 2: Open the Session and Introduce the Session Topic

After briefly checking in with the group, introduce the concept of managing stress. Point out that one of the reasons it can be hard to ignore cravings and turn down offers is that the body, mind, and emotions can "get in the way." It can also be especially difficult to avoid using alcohol or other drugs when feeling stressed.

Ask the group for examples of times when their stress affected their behavior. These examples can involve positive emotions (such as happiness, pride, excitement), or negative emotions (such as anger, fear, sadness). Next, emphasize that everyone at one point or another has managed their stress, whether they have realized it or not. Provide examples of such situations and discuss them with the group. Some examples include ignoring an insult, walking away from a fight, getting out of bed even when really depressed, or counting to 10 when angry.

Explain that biology teaches that no being can exist in two states at once. Thus, a person cannot be tense while simultaneously relaxed and calm—it is physiologically impossible. That is the basis for relaxation techniques: By relaxing both the body and the mind, people are able to manage stress without resorting to negative behaviors.

Step 3: Lead the Group through Part I of "Relaxation Scripts"—"Muscle Relaxation"

Point out to the group that relaxation takes practice; it does not come naturally to everyone. Explain that you will be leading some relaxation exercises in which group members close their eyes and imagine different situations. If you have never facilitated relaxation exercises, just remember that the goal is to help the group *relax*. So, when leading the exercises, speak in a soothing but natural voice, a little slower than usual, and pause where indicated.

Begin by having the group members find a comfortable position in which to sit (no lying down because this encourages sleep!), close their eyes, and focus on your voice. Read the "Muscle Relaxation" script (Figure A/M-3.1) aloud slowly (you should read the script rather than distributing it). Watch the group members as you do so, paying particular attention to clients who do not seem to be relaxing (you should be able to notice based on their body language). When you have finished, discuss this activity with group members. Were they able to relax? Did anything change during the exercise (mood, tenseness)? Can the group members tell a difference?

Step 4: Lead the Group through Part II of "Relaxation Scripts"—"Marbles and Paint"

Tell group members that some relaxation exercises are helpful when they are having trouble calming down or thinking clearly; the next exercise is a good example of this. Have group members close their eyes. Slowly read the "Marbles and Paint" script (Figure A/M-3.1) aloud. When you have finished, discuss this activity with the group. Were group members able to picture the marbles in their mind? Did this help clear their minds?

Step 5: Close the Session

Point out that you have demonstrated two examples of ways to manage stress, but there are many other tools clients can use. One such tool is meditation. Explain that meditation is one way that people relax on a regular basis. Although it is similar to muscle relaxation, it focuses more on calming the mind *as well as* the body. Also, this technique can help people think more clearly by filtering out distractions. Distribute the "Meditation" handout (A/M-3.1) and suggest that the effects of this tool are cumulative. By practicing daily, people can develop the skills to relax and stay calm even in the most difficult situations.

Summarize the session, stressing that the relaxation tools are not designed to *solve* problems but to help control stress and avoid resorting to negative behaviors. Point out that using these techniques to ignore situations will *not* be helpful; people can relax in stressful situations, so that they will make rational decisions rather than impulsive, poor choices. Check in with group members. Ask them to choose one technique and practice it daily between now and the next session.

STEP-BY-STEP SESSION TASKS

Step 1: Open the session and check in with group members (approximately 10 minutes).

Step 2: Introduce the session topic: Managing stress (approximately 10 minutes).

- Ask group members to give examples of times when stressful situations (positive or negative) affected their behavior.
- Provide and discuss several examples of situations in which group members might have managed their stress response without even realizing it.
- Discuss the relationship between stress and the body, thoughts, and emotions.
- Explain that relaxation is one way to manage stress.

Part I: Muscle Relaxation

We are going to help your body to relax, but we will do this one part at a time. First, pay attention to your breathing. Take long . . . slow . . . deep breaths—fill up your entire chest—hold that breath . . . now release. Again—take a deep breath . . . hold it . . . now release. Keep breathing slowly . . . Now we will begin relaxing with your feet—pay close attention to how your toes are feeling. Slowly begin to relax each toe: start your left foot and work your way across your right foot. Count to yourself as you relax each toe . . . 1 . . . 2 . . . 3 . . . 4 . . . 5 . . . 6 . . . 7 . . . 8 . . . 9 . . . 10. (*pause*)

Now, pay attention to your ankles. Slowly rotate each ankle—first the right . . . and now the left. Let the tension leave your ankles, then rest them on the floor. Let the floor support your feet—don't try to hold them up; let all of your weight go into the floor.

Focus on your breathing. Take a deep breath . . . hold it . . . and now release. How are your calves feeling? Slowly relax your left calf—let all the tension go. Now, relax your right calf—your legs are feeling lighter and lighter as the tension disappears.

Moving up, pay attention to your thighs—are they weighted down and heavy? Slowly relax your right thigh . . . take a deep breath . . . exhale. Now relax your left thigh. . . . The weight is gone from your legs.

Next, pay attention to your stomach. Slowly relax your stomach . . . . Let the tension leave your body. Think about your breathing. Take a deep breath . . . hold it . . . and release. Feel your chest move with each breath. With each breath more tension and stress leave your body. Relax your chest muscles after each breath—it is getting easier to breath slowly.

Pay attention to your shoulders—are they tense? Slowly release the tightness in your shoulders. Feel your left shoulder—move your left arm in a circular motion . . . now your right. Pay attention to your upper arm. Relax your right muscle. . . . Now relax your left upper arm. . . . Your shoulders are light and relaxed.

Pay attention to your lower arms. Loosen the tension in your lower left arm. . . . Relax up your lower right arm . . . let go of the tension. Feel your wrists . . . Slowly rotate your left wrist . . . now your right. Let the tension leave your wrists . . . your hands are light—rest them on the floor or your legs.

Pay attention to your hands. One by one relax your fingers. Start with the left hand . . . work your way to your right hand. Your hands are relaxed.

Pay attention to your back. Arch your back and let your muscles stretch out . . . now release and return to your original position. Slowly roll your neck around . . . and around again. Your head is light and your neck is relaxed. Pay attention to your face. Start with your forehead and relax each muscle . . . your cheeks, your mouth, your chin.

Pay attention to your body—if you feel a muscle that is tense, release it and relax. You are totally relaxed and the stress is gone from your body.

Part II: Marbles and Paint

Start to slow your mind down . . . imagine that your mind is a huge glass jar, and you can see everything going on inside it. Now imagine that every thought you are having is a colored marble rolling around the jar; there are so many colors it is almost blinding.

Slowly bring the marbles to a complete stop . . . they slow down and finally rest on the bottom of the jar. The jar is full of marbles of every color . . . red . . . orange . . . yellow . . . green . . . blue . . . purple

(continued)

FIGURE A/M-3.1. Relaxation Scripts. "Marbles and Paint" from T. Linder (personal communication, 1995). Reprinted by permission.

. . . white . . . black . . . and every color in between. One by one, begin to take the marbles out of the jar . . . start with the marbles on top, and work your way down to the very last marble. Place the marbles in a basket that is sitting next to the jar. When the jar is empty, look at the basket.

The marbles have started to blend together . . . they form a beautiful rainbow of color, with stripes here and there of various shades. You stir the colors together, and pour the paint out of the basket into the stream that you are standing next to. The water surrounds the rainbow of color—and then it is gone.

Look back at the jar—it is empty, quiet, and at rest.

FIGURE A/M 3.1. (*cont.*)

Step 3: Lead the group through Part I of "Relaxation Scripts"—"Muscle Relaxation" (Figure A/M-3.1) (approximately 15–20 minutes).

- Point out that relaxation takes practice, and that you will be practicing two exercises today.

- Have group members sit comfortably, close their eyes, and focus on your voice.

- Slowly read Part I aloud, pausing between paragraphs.

- Discuss this activity.

Step 4: Lead the group through Part II of "Meditation"—"Marbles and Paint" (Figure A/M-3.1) (approximately 15 minutes).

- Ask clients to close their eyes and listen to your voice.

- Slowly read Part II aloud.

- Discuss this activity.

Step 5: Close the session (approximately 10 minutes).

- Explain that one other tool to manage stress is through the use of meditation. Distribute the "Relaxation Scripts" handout (A/M-3.1).

- Summarize the session.

- Emphasize that these techniques do not *solve* problems but can help control thoughts and emotions so that people can act more in line with their intentions.

- Briefly check in with clients.

- Ask clients to choose one of the three techniques and practice it daily between now and the next session.

MEDITATION

Getting Ready

The first step in meditation is to make sure that your posture is good. (With meditation you are not only training your mind but also your body). You can sit either on the floor, using a cushion, or in a chair with your feet touching the floor. Following these guidelines will allow your breath to flow more easily and deeply:

- Back straight
- Shoulders relaxed
- Head upright
- Chin tilted down

- Eyes only partially closed and gaze softened
- Hands resting lightly on the legs

In general, begin with meditating 20 minutes at a time—you can begin with doing this once a day, twice a day if possible. It usually takes 15–20 minutes to settle the mind, so the optimal session lasts from 20–35 minutes. Try to choose times to meditate when you are not particularly tired.

What to Do

Begin by breathing deep into your abdomen. (Many times, people tend to breathe shallow and into their chest. Breathe quietly through your nose with your mouth closed.) Notice the rise and fall of your abdomen. Sit quietly, paying attention to your breathing (in . . . out . . . in . . . out). When you notice distracting thoughts arising (and they will), gently return to focusing on your breathing. Do not become frustrated with yourself for thinking of other things, but do not pursue those thoughts, either.

Sometimes it is helpful to use counting as a means of focusing. On the first inhale count "1," then exhale on "2" . . . inhale on "3" . . . exhale on "4," and so on, until you reach "10." If you find yourself losing count or having a distracting thought, begin again at "1." Let your thoughts easily come and go, like clouds changing shapes or moving across the sky. Do not cling to them—let them go. Then return to an awareness of the present moment by focusing on your breathing.

As you calm your mind, it is helpful to calm the body. Try to sit as still as possible while you meditate. You might find that different parts of your body begin to ache from sitting still. There are several ways to deal with these discomforts: first, just notice the ache and focus on your breathing again (the ache may disappear); second, observe the ache, breathe into it, and explore it; finally, if the discomfort becomes too great, slowly shift to a more comfortable position.

A/M SESSION 4

Rewarding My Successes

CHANGE PROCESS OBJECTIVE: REINFORCEMENT MANAGEMENT

RATIONALE

Reinforcement management involves rewarding positive behavior changes; these can take the form of actual "rewards" or may simply be the positive consequences resulting from behaviors that prevent alcohol or drug use. This session begins to use this change process by stressing the importance of rewarding even the smallest changes. By identifying potential rewards, clients can learn to reward themselves when they take a positive step toward behavior change.

CONTENT OBJECTIVES

Clients understand the importance of rewarding positive behavior.
Clients identify recent accomplishments.
Clients brainstorm examples of ways to reward positive behaviors.

MATERIALS REQUIRED

Copies of the "Rewarding My Successes" handout (A/M-4.1) for distribution to each group member

SESSION SUMMARY

The facilitator explains that, often, clients neither acknowledge nor reward the "small" steps that lead to behavior change and emphasizes that behaviors that are rewarded (or

146

"reinforced") tend to occur again. Clients identify past accomplishments in order to practice recognizing successes, and they identify rewards that they can begin to implement following positive steps toward behavior change or maintenance.

IMPLEMENTATION

Clients often have difficulty acknowledging when they make positive steps toward behavior change. Instead, they tend to dwell on the negative. This may be due, in part, to years of looking "down" on themselves as a result of their substance use, although many people, in general, have difficulty in acknowledging the "good things" that they accomplish. In today's session, emphasize the importance of clients' recognition of the positive steps they take toward behavior change, as well as reinforcement of those steps with rewards.

Steps 1 and 2: Open the Session and Introduce the Topic

Briefly check in with the group and introduce the topic by explaining that any behavior is comprised of several small steps. For instance, if you wanted to cook a meal, you would first need to buy food with which to cook. You would have to go to the grocery store, select your items, pay for the groceries, go back home, and complete the steps required to cook the food. Many times, people become so focused on the end result (i.e., having a meal to eat) that they lose sight of the steps they had to complete in order to achieve the result (i.e., going to the store, purchasing groceries, following a recipe).

Point out that clients who have stopped using alcohol or other drugs also tend to focus on the end result (abstinence from substance use) rather than acknowledging the numerous "small" steps or successes that helped them become alcohol- and drug-free.

Step 3: Identify Recent Successes

Ask clients to think about and share a few successes that they have accomplished during the past 6 months. These successes could be as "small," such as simply getting out of bed in the morning with a good attitude, or as "large" as helping someone else quit using alcohol or drugs. Model reinforcement skills by congratulating each client on these accomplishments. Discuss these successes with the group using questions similar to the following:

- "Were there any rewards that followed these successes?"
- "If so, did someone else do the rewarding or did you initiate it yourself?"
- "If not, what were the barriers to rewards after your success?"

(*Note.* You may need to prompt some clients who are unable to think of any successes. Some suggestions could be attending this group, supporting other group members, realizing that they have a substance use problem, removing drugs or alcohol from their home, or avoiding people or places that might encourage substance use.)

Step 4: Generate Ideas for Self-Rewards

Point out that clients may have had difficulty in recognizing achievements related to their substance use. In that case, it is likely they have not made a priority of rewarding themselves for these successes along the way. Explain that research shows that behaviors that are rewarded, or "reinforced," tend to reoccur and often become habitual. Emphasize that as the clients continue working to avoid alcohol and other drug use, it will be important for them to reward their efforts.

Break the group into pairs and distribute the "Rewarding My Successes" handout (A/M-4.1). Have the pairs discuss and write down as many rewarding things as they can think of (no matter how unrealistic they might sound). Point out that what is a reward for one person may not necessarily be a reward for someone else. Also emphasize that not all rewards cost money, and some do not even involve objects—a reward can be as simple as taking a walk at sunset. It is also important for group members to remember that we often get rewarded by others; have them write down rewards they might receive from other sources as well. Give some examples to the pairs (such as the following) and circulate among the pairs giving assistance as needed:

- Eating a favorite food
- Spending time with a friend
- Taking a hot bath
- Watching a movie
- Playing a sport or exercising
- Taking time to read a book or magazine
- Buying yourself a present

Step 5: Discuss the Activity

Bring the group back together, and have the pairs share the rewards they wrote down on their handouts. Have clients add to their lists any ideas other pairs describe that they appreciate as well. Facilitate a discussion regarding these ideas.

Step 6: Close the Session

Check in with the group and summarize the session by emphasizing the importance of rewarding even the smallest step toward making or maintaining behavior change. Point out that clients have worked hard to "get where they are" in terms of reducing their substance use—they deserve rewards! Ask them to choose three of the rewards on their list and implement them regularly over the next month, whenever they take steps to remain alcohol and/or drug-free.

STEP-BY-STEP SESSION TASKS

Step 1: Open the session and check in with the group (approximately 10 minutes).

Step 2: Introduce the topic: Rewarding my successes (approximately 5 minutes).

- Explain that any behavior is comprised of small steps.
- Point out that, many times, people tend to become so focused on an end result that they forget about the steps that lead them to that result.
- Explain that some clients tend to focus on their abstinence rather than acknowledging the small steps they took to become alcohol- and/or drug-free.

Step 3: Identify recent successes (approximately 10 minutes).

- Have clients think about and share examples of successes they have had during the past 6 months.
- Model reinforcement skills by congratulating clients on these accomplishments.
- Assist clients who have difficulty remembering successes.
- Facilitate a discussion regarding these successes and rewards.

Step 4: Generate ideas for self-rewards (approximately 20 minutes).

- Point out the importance of not only recognizing successes but also rewarding them.
- Explain that behaviors that are rewarded are more likely to occur again.
- Break the groups into pairs.
- Distribute the "Rewarding My Successes" handout (A/M-4.1).
- Have the pairs generate ideas for things that would be rewarding to them.
- Emphasize that rewards do not have to involve money or objects, may differ from one person to another, and can be initiated by the clients themselves or other people.
- Give a few examples of rewards and circulate among the pairs, offering assistance as needed.

Step 5: Discuss the activity (approximately 10 minutes).

- Bring the group back together.
- Have the pairs share the ideas they wrote down.
- Have clients write down any additional rewards they might appreciate as the pairs share their lists.
- Discuss these ideas for rewards with the group.

Step 6: Close the session (approximately 5 minutes).

- Briefly check in with the group.
- Summarize the session.
- Affirm clients for their participation

REWARDING MY SUCCESSES

Things I can do to reward myself when I succeed in avoiding alcohol or other drug use:

Effective Communication

CHANGE PROCESS OBJECTIVES: COUNTERCONDITIONING, REINFORCEMENT MANAGEMENT

RATIONALE

In a situation where it is difficult to alter or avoid triggers to use, another effective strategy is for clients to alter *their responses* to the cues. This change process of *counterconditioning* involves substituting healthy behaviors for unhealthy responses. The change process of *reinforcement management* involves rewarding positive behavior changes.

This session combines these two processes of change. When interacting with others, it can be very difficult for clients to alter or avoid triggers that involve the other person (i.e., employ stimulus control). When this happens, it is useful to use counterconditioning instead, and alter our *responses* to the triggers. This session assists clients in learning how to do that through the use of effective communication skills. Experiencing a positive result due to effective communication reinforces the likelihood that clients will continue to use these skills in future interactions.

CONTENT OBJECTIVES

Clients learn three styles of communication (passive, aggressive, and assertive).
Clients determine their typical ways of communicating with others.
Clients learn tools to communicate effectively.

MATERIALS REQUIRED

Chalkboard or flipchart.
Copies of the following for distribution to each group member: "Effective Communication" handout (A/M-5.1)

SESSION SUMMARY

The group discusses passive, aggressive, and assertive communication styles. The facilitator reviews "tips" for effective communication. Group members split up into pairs and role-play all three types of responses, then discuss which of the three scenarios are the most successful/healthy.

IMPLEMENTATION

Even though clients may be aware that being offered alcohol or drugs places them at high risk of relapse, it is often hard for them simply to avoid situations where offers might be made. It may be necessary that clients express themselves clearly to avoid relapse. In today's session, you will discuss the difference between *passive*, *aggressive*, and *assertive* communication. You will also teach the clients a three-step technique to help them respond using effective communication skills.

Steps 1 and 2: Open the Session and Introduce the Topic

Explain that how we communicate often dictates how others respond to us. Describe the three main styles of communication: aggressive, passive, and assertive.

- People who communicate *passively* tend to give up their rights if there seems to be a conflict between what they want and what someone else wants. Many times, they "bottle up" their emotions and do not let others know what they are feeling and thinking. An example of a passive response is when a person is upset and does not communicate that to others. They often "go along" just to avoid conflict.
- People who communicate *aggressively* try to protect their own rights, but in doing so, they ignore the rights and feelings of others. Although they may get what they want in the short term, the long-term effects of aggressiveness are often negative. Aggressive people often make others angry or hurt their feelings by disregarding their needs. An example of an aggressive response is when a person loudly pushes his or her agenda regardless of what other people want.
- People who communicate *assertively* decide what it is they need, clearly state their feelings and opinions, and request directly the changes that they would like from others. Assertive people do this without directing threats, demands, or negative statements at others. For example, in an assertive response, a person makes his or her needs known in a way that doesn't discount other people's feelings.

Give examples of each of these approaches to communication and write them on a chalkboard or flipchart. Explain that all of us, at one time or another, have used each of these three types of communication. However, an assertive response is helpful and more likely to send a message that is closer to what the person actually intends, and the listener is more likely to "hear" the message more clearly.

Step 3: Determine Typical Ways Clients Communicate with Others

Point out that most people usually communicate in a certain way; however, this can change on any given day or at any moment (based on situation, interaction, mood, physical health, etc.). Ask the group members how they think they usually communicate with others.

Distribute the "Effective Communication" handout (A/M-5.1). Read the scenario in Part I aloud. Ask the clients how they would typically respond in this situation, and ask them to discuss their thoughts. Explain that some people might respond in a passive way, taking the blame and suffering the consequences. Others might respond in an aggressive way, yelling that this "is not fair" and blaming someone else. Finally, still others might respond assertively, calmly telling the manager, for example, that they did not take the money and explaining that they have receipts to prove it.

Step 4: Describe Tools to Communicate Assertively

Explain that you will be teaching a few tools to help clients communicate in effective ways. Point out that instead of focusing on what the other person is doing, assertive communication focuses on *their own reactions* to that behavior. One way to do this is to start sentences with the word "I" instead of "you." When we begin a statement with "you," it often places blame on the other person; starting with "I" helps us take responsibility for our behavior, thoughts, and feelings. For example, notice the difference between "I get frustrated when I feel like you do not listen to me" and "You never listen to what I say."

Another way to use effective communication skills is to think of assertive messages as having three parts: describing the behavior, describing your feelings/reactions, and describing what you want to see happen. Read Part II of the "Effective Communication" handout (A/M-5.1) aloud. Then, refer back to the scenario in Part I. Give an example of how Tom might have responded assertively (something like "I understand that you think I took the money, and I am frustrated that you do not trust me. I would like you to check my receipts against the cash box to see that I did not take the money.").

Read Part III ("tips") aloud and ask if any members have additional suggestions from their experiences.

Step 5: Close the Session

Summarize the session by pointing out the advantages of using effective communication (i.e., positive consequences, respect, more control). Remind the group that when they choose to use effective communication skills, they are not only respecting themselves but also, they are respecting the other person. Check in with members to address any remaining issues and ask clients to practice using effective communication a few times each week.

STEP-BY-STEP SESSION TASKS

Step 1: Open the session and check in with group members (approximately 10 minutes).

Step 2: Introduce the session topic: Effective communication (approximately 10 minutes).

- Describe the three main styles of communication.
- Discuss and write examples of each on the chalkboard/flipchart.
- Explain that responses are based on underlying thoughts and feelings, and that each interaction has consequences.

Step 3: Determine typical ways clients communicate with others (approximately 10 minutes).

- Point out that most people typically communicate a certain way, but this can vary depending on circumstances.
- Distribute the "Effective Communication" handout (A/M-5.1).
- Read the scenario in Part I aloud.
- Have group members discuss how they would typically respond, and give examples of passive, aggressive, and assertive responses.

Step 4: Describe tools to communicate effectively (approximately 20 minutes).

- Point out that instead of focusing on what the other person is doing to them, effective communication focuses *on their own reactions* to that behavior.
- Explain the use of "I" statements.
- Read Part II of "Effective Communication" aloud.
- Refer to the scenario in Part I and give an example of how Tom might have responded assertively, using the technique in Part II.
- Read Part III of "Effective Communication" aloud.

Step 5: Close the session (approximately 10 minutes).

- Summarize the session and check in with group members.
- Ask group members to practice communicating effectively a few times each day, between now and the next session.

EFFECTIVE COMMUNICATION

Part I: For Example . . .

Tom had been working at this job for quite some time. Part of his job was to be in charge of the cash box. Someone started a rumor that he was stealing money, and his boss heard the rumor. The next day, his boss (who was very angry) yelled at him, accusing him of stealing.

What would you say?

Part II: Three Steps to Effective Communication

1. **Describe the behavior**—Tell the person your perception of what he or she is doing. Be sure you are describing the behaviors and not calling the other person names or making accusations.
2. **Describe your feelings or reactions**—Tell the person how you feel about the behavior, or how it affects you. For example, "I feel mad because" . . .
3. **Describe what you want to see happen**—Tell the person what you would like for him or her to do. Remember to use specific descriptions that focus on the behavior rather than putting the other person down.

Part III: Here are a few tips to help you communicate effectively!

- Speak in a clear, firm, voice.
- Make direct eye contact.
- Use statements that begin with "I."
- Don't feel guilty!
- Suggest alternatives.
- Avoid excuses or vague answers.
- Be direct and clear.
- "No" is enough—you don't have to explain your reasons.
- Be aware of body language.

Part II is adapted from Huszti (1997). Part III is adapted from Monti, Abrams, Kadden, and Cooney (1989). Copyright 1989 by The Guilford Press. Reprinted in Velasquez, Maurer, Crouch, and DiClemente (2001). Copyright by The Guilford Press. Permission to photocopy this handout is granted to purchasers of this book for personal use only (see copyright page for details).

Effective Refusals

CHANGE PROCESS OBJECTIVES:
COUNTERCONDITIONING, REINFORCEMENT MANAGEMENT

RATIONALE

In a situation where it is difficult to alter or avoid triggers, another effective strategy is for clients to alter *their responses* to the triggers. This change process of *counterconditioning* involves substitution of healthy for unhealthy responses. The change process of *reinforcement management* involves rewarding positive behavior changes.

As does the previous session, this one combines these two processes of change. It builds on the effective communication tools presented in A/M Session 5. This session is designed to help clients learn how to change (or *countercondition*) their responses to the trigger of being offered alcohol or another drug through the use of refusal skills. After successfully refusing an offer, the likelihood that clients will refuse in the future is strengthened when clients' refusal skills are *reinforced*.

CONTENT OBJECTIVES

Clients think of people who currently use and might offer them alcohol or drugs. Clients practice using refusal skills to decline offers to use.

MATERIALS REQUIRED

Copies of the "Practicing Refusals" handout (A/M-6.1) for distribution to each group member

SESSION SUMMARY

The facilitator has group members think of times when they successfully refused offers to use alcohol/drugs. The group discusses and writes down examples of realistic offers to use. The facilitator conducts a role play in which clients attempt to "persuade" a partner into having a drink or a drug. The partner is only allowed to say "no" and uses his or her body language and intonation to help express the refusal effectively.

IMPLEMENTATION

In working with clients, many times we have seen how difficult it can be for them—even when simply doing an exercise—to refuse an offer. In fact, their body language often demonstrates their reluctance to say "no." For instance, they may tend to draw inward with shoulders slumped and make little eye contact, and often seem nervous or unsure. Because they do not appear comfortable or confident, their refusal loses its believability, in some ways, they make themselves easy targets for persistent offers. It appears as though they might "give in" if badgered long enough.

Because clients may be unable to avoid interacting with people who currently use and make offers of alcohol or other drugs, it is important to assist them in gaining the skills to communicate clearly their intention to remain substance-free. This session focuses on how clients can effectively "turn down" a drink or drug when it is offered to them. A helpful strategy in doing so is to identify the times in which offers to use are most likely to occur and then practice saying "no" to the offers. By being aware ahead of time, clients have the opportunity to be more prepared when an offer does arise.

Steps 1 and 2: Open the Session and Introduce the Session Topic

Check in with the group and introduce the topic by pointing out that it can be difficult to avoid people who are using alcohol or other drugs. Many times, these current users make offers to "join in" to people who have stopping using alcohol or drugs. This can be an awkward and quite tempting situation for clients who have not anticipated such a blatant temptation. Point out that a helpful strategy for refusing offers is to identify the times in which offers to use are most likely to occur and practice saying "no" to those offers.

Step 3: Identify Current Users

Ask group members to think about the people with whom they currently interact who use alcohol or drugs. It may help the group in identifying these current users to give prompts such as "What about your family members, friends, coworkers, neighbors?" and so on. Facilitate a group discussion about the situations surrounding these relationships. Are they tempted to "join in" when they see others using? How often do these current users offer alcohol or other drugs to the clients? Explain that in these relationships, it may be difficult to avoid being around alcohol or drug use, and it may be even *more* difficult to avoid an offer to use. Ask if any group members have successfully turned down an offer to use. If they have, ask them to share with the group how they did this.

Step 4: Practice Refusing Offers to Use

Explain that one way to prepare clients for a situation is to pretend that it is actually happening and practice how they would respond. This technique can be very effective and is called *role playing*. By putting themselves in a "role," they can see how it would feel to be in specific situations and to try different ways of responding.

Divide the group into pairs and distribute the "Practicing Refusals" handout (A/M-6.1). Read the instructions for each role aloud and answer any questions. Have the pairs begin the role plays. Walk among them and make sure that clients in the refusing role respond only with the single word "no." Coach them as needed, pointing out that they need to relax, sit upright, maintain eye contact, and so on, to embody effectively their refusal. Help clients also be aware of the tone and inflection in their voice. Allow the role plays to continue for 3 minutes. Then, have the clients switch roles (those who made the offer the first time will now be refusing, and those who just "refused" will now make the offers). Allow the pairs to do this second role play for 3 minutes, walking among the pairs and coaching as before.

Step 5: Discuss the Role Plays

When the pairs have finished, discuss this activity with the group using the questions for discussion from the "Practicing Refusals" handout (A/M-6.1). How was this refusal different from their refusals in the past (besides in the role play)? What are the benefits of using this exercise to turn down an offer? Explain to clients that it can be very rewarding to use this exercise effectively. Each time they are able to do this successfully, their confidence to use refusal skills in future situations is increased.

Step 6: Close the Session

Explain that this exercise demonstrates how one can effectively learn to refuse offers to use substances. Often, when we try to refuse an offer, we feel that we have to provide a reason. We all have had the experience of telling someone "no" and having them ask "why," asking us to give a reason. But we don't have to provide others with a reason; saying "no" can be enough. Giving a reason opens the door to others to "counter" the argument. They will often try to talk us out of our point of view, to persuade, to disagree, and so on. Saying only the word "no" can help close the door to these counterarguments. Spoken with authority and confident body language, clients can usually put an end to the request immediately.

Briefly check in with the group, summarize the session, and tell the clients that it will be helpful to practice these skills in order to become more comfortable in turning down offers to use alcohol or other drugs. Also ask group members to be aware of their own body language when they turn down offers to use.

STEP-BY-STEP SESSION TASKS

Step 1: Open the session (approximately 10 minutes).

- Brief check in with group members.
- Review assertive communication from A/M Session 5.

Step 2: Introduce the session topic: Refusal skills (approximately 10 minutes).

Step 3: Identify current users (approximately 10 minutes).

- Ask group members to think about the people with whom they currently interact who use alcohol or drugs.
- Facilitate a group discussion about the situations surrounding relationships, without using anyone's real name. How much of a trigger is the person, the usual situation?.
- Explain that clients may not always be able to *avoid* offers to use.
- Ask about the times that they have successfully turned down offers to use alcohol or other drugs.

Step 4: Practice using refusal skills to decline offers (approximately 10 minutes).

- Explain the concept of role play.
- Divide the group into pairs, distribute the "Practicing Refusals" handout (A/M-6.1) and read the instructions.
- Have one partner in each pair be the person making an offer to drink or use drugs; have the other decline the offer by saying *only* the word "no." This is the only response that should be used in this exercise, not other words or phrases that are typically used when declining offers.
- Have members of the pairs switch roles. Repeat the role plays.
- Walk among the pairs, coaching the partner who is saying "no" on how effectively to embody his or her refusal. This is done by suggesting that clients relax, use confident body language, speak with authority, and so on.

Step 5: Discuss the role plays (approximately 15 minutes).

- Have each pair share their experience of the role play.
- Discuss this activity using the prompts in the "Practicing Refusals" handout (A/M-6.1).

Step 6: Close the session (approximately 5 minutes).

- Summarize the session.
- Affirm members for the progress they have made.
- Check in with group members.

PRACTICING REFUSALS

This exercise is designed to help you improve your ability to refuse offers to drink or use drugs.

For the **person making the offer:** Your job is to try for a full 3 minutes to persuade the other person to take a drink. Short of physical force, you are to entice, cajole, beg, plead, implore, manipulate, and/or guilt-trip the other person. You are to say whatever you need to in order to be successful. Don't take "no" for an answer! Don't give up.

Your questions for discussion:

What was your partner's body language telling you?

Did it seem that your partner really meant "no"?

For the **person refusing the drink or drug:** The **only** thing you may say during this entire 3-minute period is "no." You may not provide reasons, excuses, explanations—**nothing** that will give the other person an opportunity to counter with stronger arguments. "No" really is enough of a reason. You can say "no" and not necessarily sound rude or impolite. Use your body language and the tone of your voice to help you say "no."

Your questions for discussion:

How did it feel to say "no"?

Did you doubt your ability to keep saying "no"?

What were your thoughts as you were trying to refuse?

What emotions did you experience?

What did you notice in your body?

Managing Criticism

CHANGE PROCESS OBJECTIVES:
COUNTERCONDITIONING, REINFORCEMENT MANAGEMENT

RATIONALE

This session combines these two processes of change: *counterconditioning* and *reinforcement management*. Often, conflict with others functions as a stimulus to use alcohol or other drugs, and it often begins with the expression of criticism. This session helps clients learn how to substitute more appropriate ways of handling criticism than conflict and substance use. Upon successfully using skills for giving and receiving criticism from others, clients' interpersonal skills are reinforced, and they will be more likely to handle criticism more appropriately in the future.

CONTENT OBJECTIVES

Clients learn how to receive criticism appropriately from others.
Clients learn techniques to give constructive effectively criticism to others.

MATERIALS REQUIRED

Copies of the "Managing Criticism" handout (A/M-7.1) for distribution to each group member

SESSION SUMMARY

Clients will discuss the fact that expression of criticism often ignites conflict, and that conflict with others can lead to frustration, anger, and temptations to use. The group will generate ideas about how to handle criticism appropriately, as well as how to give feedback effectively to others in ways less likely to escalate conflict.

IMPLEMENTATION

Interpersonal conflicts, and the resulting anger and negative feelings they elicit, can result in high-risk situations for "slips." This session helps clients learn to use effective communication skills to deal with expressions of criticism, and the anger and conflict that often result. Since criticism can generate conflict and is often viewed as a negative or unpleasant event, an important goal of this session is to learn to present and receive feedback, or criticism, in a *constructive* way that will lead to positive results for all parties involved.

Steps 1 and 2: Open the Session and Introduce the Topic

Briefly check in with the group. Introduce the topic by pointing out that everyone encounters situations where others make critical statements or give feedback that is perceived as being critical. One of the most difficult things to do when interacting with others is to receive feedback gracefully. Feedback from others can shake your confidence and leave you feeling upset and angry, especially if the feedback is expressed with hostility and aggression. For many people, these negative emotions lead to strong temptations to use alcohol or other drugs. However, feedback can actually provide a valuable opportunity to learn things about yourself and how you affect others.

Step 3: Generate Ideas about Receiving Criticism Effectively

Facilitate a group discussion about feedback by asking questions such as the following:

- "Can you remember an example of a time when someone confronted you and it seemed to 'clear the air'?"
- "Have there been other times when relationships 'went downhill' after feedback was given?"
- "Were there differences in the way that things were handled in these different situations?"

Suggest to the clients that being able to receive feedback effectively can reduce conflicts and the likelihood of a slip. Distribute the "Managing Criticism" handout (A/M-7.1) to each group member. Read each of the suggestions in Part I aloud, pointing out how these can be helpful in avoiding negative interactions with others. Have clients add any suggestions they might have to the handout.

Step 4: Generate Ideas about How to Give Criticism Appropriately

Discuss with the group examples of situations in which it is necessary to give feedback to another person in order to resolve a conflict (e.g., if a coworker is not doing his or her job and you have to "pick up the slack"). Help the clients understand that there are effective ways to do this and still maintain a working relationship with the other person. In fact, in some situations, giving appropriate feedback can strengthen the relationship if done constructively. Facilitate a group discussion, asking questions such as the following:

- "How could learning to use constructive feedback be helpful when you are frustrated with other people?"
- "Can you remember a situation in which you confronted another person about his or her behavior? How did that interaction end?"
- "Have there been times when a situation has worsened because you did *not* confront someone?"
- "Are there times when it is better not to confront another person about behavior that is causing you problems?"

Read Part II of the "Managing Criticism" handout (A/M-7.1). Have clients discuss these suggestions and also write down any additional suggestions they might have about giving constructive feedback.

Step 5: Close the Session

Briefly check in with the group and summarize the session by emphasizing the importance of respecting others during potentially frustrating interactions. Emphasize that although clients are now familiar with techniques to give and receive feedback appropriately, most people outside of the group struggle with confrontation. It may be unrealistic to expect to receive appropriate feedback or healthy responses to feedback that they give others. Clients may find it helpful to use relaxation techniques or to take time to "cool off" in order better to handle frustrations that might occur as a result of interpersonal conflict.

STEP-BY-STEP SESSION TASKS

Step 1: Open the session and check-in with the group (approximately 10 minutes).

Step 2: Introduce the topic: Managing criticism (approximately 10 minutes).

Step 3: Generate ideas about effective ways to receive feedback (approximately 15 minutes).

- Discuss situations in the past where feedback was handled well, and those in which it negatively affected the relationship.

- Explain that by learning to receive feedback effectively, clients can better avoid conflict and reduce the likelihood of a slip.
- Distribute the "Managing Criticism" handout (A/M-7.1).
- Read the suggestions in Part I aloud.
- Discuss these and have clients write down any further suggestions they might have.

Step 4: Generate ideas about how to give feedback appropriately (approximately 15 minutes).

- Point out that many clients are tempted to use alcohol or other drugs when they are frustrated due to a conflict with someone.
- Explain that there are effective ways to give feedback and keep a positive relationship with the other person.
- Discuss the experiences the group has had with giving feedback to someone else.
- Read the suggestions in Part II of the "Managing Criticism" handout (A/M-7.1) aloud.
- Discuss these and have clients add any further suggestions they may have.

Step 5: Close the session (approximately 10 minutes).

- Briefly check in with the clients.
- Summarize the session.

MANAGING CRITICISM

Part I: Receiving Feedback—The strategies listed below can help you appropriately handle the situation when someone confronts you, regardless of whether the feedback is *constructive* or *destructive*.

- **Keep cool: Avoid escalation**—Make a conscious effort to relax by using relaxation techniques. If the other person is *very* upset, and you feel yourself "losing it," try explaining that you want to discuss the issues, but only after you have both calmed down and you can think more clearly.
- **Listen: Show that you want to understand**—Let the other person have his or her say without interrupting; hear him or her out. Try summarizing what he or she said by saying: "I thought I heard you say _____. Is that right?" This helps to clarify what he or she is saying and shows that you are trying to listen well.
- **Apologize: Correct misunderstandings**—Try to determine if there has been some misunderstanding. If you are the one mistaken, apologize and, if appropriate, discuss what steps you can take to "put things right."

Part II: Giving Feedback—The strategies listed below can help you appropriately handle the situation when you need to confront someone else.

- **Stay calm**—Try not to challenge anyone about his or her behavior if you are feeling very angry. You need to be in control to be constructive and to choose your words carefully; if you are not, you may say things that you will regret.
- **Choose the right time and place**—Decide when it is the right time and place. Many times, it is not appropriate to confront someone when others are around; this can be embarrassing for everyone.
- **Check out misunderstandings**—Before confronting someone, make sure to check that there has been no misunderstanding. This gives you the chance to back down gracefully if the mistake is your own, and gives the other person the chance to apologize if the mistake is his or hers.
- **Don't blame**—If there is no misunderstanding but the other person does not understand your perspective, help him or her to see things from your point of view. Do so, making sure to focus on the behavior, not the person.
- **Use "I" language**—Use your assertive communication skills to deliver "I" messages. Focus on *your* responsibilities and needs, and the problems that arise for you as a result of the other person's behavior.

Managing Thoughts

CHANGE PROCESS OBJECTIVES: STIMULUS CONTROL, COUNTERCONDITIONING, REINFORCEMENT MANAGEMENT

RATIONALE

Today's session combines the processes of *stimulus control, counterconditioning, and reinforcement management* to teach clients how to manage and redirect thoughts that could lead to substance use. Clients can use stimulus control to alter tempting cues by *stopping* and redirecting a thought process before acting on it. By *replacing* the unhealthy thought process with healthy, substance-free thoughts and actions, clients will be utilizing counterconditioning. Finally, the positive consequence of avoiding substance use will reinforce clients' efforts to manage potentially unhealthy thoughts in the future.

CONTENT OBJECTIVES

Clients identify how thoughts can tempt one to use alcohol and other drugs.
Clients learn techniques by which to manage thoughts.

MATERIALS REQUIRED

Copies of the "Maladaptive Thoughts" handout (A/M-8.1) for distribution to each group member
Chalkboard and chalk or flipchart and markers
Pens or pencils

SESSION SUMMARY

The facilitator helps the group brainstorm and discuss examples of unhealthy thoughts (i.e., thoughts that can lead to substance use). Group members think of the last time that they used alcohol or drugs and remember the thought process that precipitated that use. Then, clients remember times in the past when they successfully managed unhealthy thoughts. The facilitator helps the group think of ways to mange and redirect thoughts, and provides tools to assist in this process.

IMPLEMENTATION

Many clients are unaware of the role that cognitions play in their lives. They may be equally unaware that a thought itself can be (and usually is) a stimulus. By helping clients recognize unhealthy thoughts as they occur, and giving them the tools to manage these thoughts, you facilitate use of the change processes of stimulus control, counterconditioning, and reinforcement management.

(*Note.* This session, while being "light" in terms of activities, is actually rich in content. Try to engage the clients in in-depth discussions and have them add suggestions from their past experiences as appropriate.)

Steps 1 and 2: Open the Session and Introduce the Topic

Begin the session by explaining that thoughts play a key role in the decisions that people make. Point out that people constantly have thoughts but sometimes do not notice them. By learning how to identify when thoughts can lead to substance use, the group will be better able to pay attention to and successfully manage them. These are often called "maladaptive" or "unhealthy" thoughts. One way to view behavior change is to see it as making a series of decisions, one after another, every day. Specifically, at some point during the thought process, people make a decision either to act on their thoughts or simply let them go. If they can recognize that they are thinking in a way that might lead to substance use, they can stop that unhealthy thought before making the decision to act.

Step 3: Noticing Maladaptive Thoughts

Explain to clients that the way we think influences how we feel and behave. It is important to pay attention to the way in which we perceive situations. Sometimes we assume a negative rather than positive style of thinking. This negative thinking can be self-fulfilling and lead to low self-esteem, depression, or anger. Clients should learn to recognize their negative thoughts and moods and to take these as signals to change the negative thinking rather than to give up and use substances. Monti, Abrams, Kadden, and Cooney (1989) suggest some skills guidelines that clients can use in changing negative thoughts.

The main steps to changing negative thinking are as follows:

• Catch yourself thinking negatively. You must learn what ways of thinking negatively you've developed over the years. And you must notice them as they are occurring. Your moods can be a sign that negative thinking is occurring. An example might be depressed mood as a result of earlier negative thinking.

• Stop the negative thinking pattern, substituting more reasonable or positive thoughts instead. Challenge and/or replace negative thoughts with those that are either neutral or positive.

Step 4: Brainstorm and Discuss Examples of Maladaptive Thoughts

Distribute the "Maladaptive Thoughts" handout (A/M-8.1). Give the example of a hot, summer day, when the thought "I'm really thirsty" might arise. Explain that another thought that might follow soon afterward could be "An ice cold beer would be great right about now!" Point out that this line of thinking could lead to memories of having cold beers when outdoors, and this could lead to strong temptations to use. Also, maladaptive thoughts are likely to occur when people have been exposed to a trigger situation (such as a party, if they are experiencing physical pain or are emotionally upset).

Have group members remember the last time that they used alcohol or other drugs. Explain that even if they were not aware of it, they had a series of thoughts that led to that substance use. Point out that the first step in addressing maladaptive thoughts is learning how to notice them when they occur. Ask clients to think for a moment about that situation and try to remember what thoughts were going through their minds. Examples might be "What's the use? I may as well have a drink," "I'll show them! I can do whatever I want to," or "I can't deal with this! Forget it—I'm going to get high."

Have group members write down these examples on Part I of the handout. When they are finished, ask: "What were these thoughts? How frequently do they occur now?" Point out that sometimes a thought in and of itself may not be tempting, but the combination of that thought with other triggers (such as certain emotions, pressure by friends, habit or routine) can prove overwhelming. What factors "pushed" these from being just thoughts into action? If the group has difficulty in remembering examples of prior thoughts, suggest that, many times, people who struggle with alcohol/drug abuse have thoughts that start with "I have to have this drink because . . . " or "I need this joint to. . . . " Emphasize the importance of clients' learning to notice their thoughts.

Step 5: Brainstorm and Discuss Ways to Manage Maladaptive Thoughts

Ask group members to think for a minute about times when they were able to "ignore" or "let go" of a thought that could have resulted in substance use. How did they do this? How were they able to "talk themselves out of" doing something that might not have been in their best interest? Write their suggestions on the chalkboard/flipchart.

Explain that there are many ways to manage automatic, harmful thoughts, and that it is important for clients to be aware of what works best for each of them. Review the following examples of ways to redirect thoughts with the group and write them on the chalkboard/flipchart:

- *Pay attention to your thoughts.* Stop before acting and concentrate on what you have been thinking. Could these thoughts "cause trouble"? What expectations do you have about the alcohol or drug use? Are these realistic expectations? What are the possible consequences of this action? If you were in a different mood, place, or time, would you be making the same decision?
- *Speak out loud.* Sometimes by actually verbalizing a thought, it is easier to recognize it as being maladaptive or irrational.
- Tell yourself to wait 30 minutes before you decide to take action.
- Do something to distract yourself.

Discuss all the suggestions written on the flipchart and have the group write any of them that they feel would help in managing thoughts on Part II of the "Maladaptive Thoughts" (A/M-8.1) handout.

Step 6: Close the Session

Summarize the session by reviewing the importance of thoughts in maintaining sobriety. Briefly check in with the group members and ask them to begin noticing their thoughts, speaking them aloud, and practicing the tools to manage harmful thoughts as they arise.

STEP-BY-STEP SESSION TASKS

Step 1: Open the session and check in with group members (approximately 5 minutes).

Step 2: Introduce the session topic: Managing thoughts (approximately 5 minutes).

Step 3: Help clients notice maladaptive thoughts (approximately 15 minutes).

- Discuss the different ways clients can perceive situations.
- Point out that patterns of negative thinking have developed over the years.
- Introduce ways to notice and replace negative thinking.

Step 4: Brainstorm and discuss examples of maladaptive thoughts (approximately 15 minutes).

- Distribute the "Maladaptive Thoughts" handout (A/M-8.1).
- Have group members remember their last use and recreate the thoughts that precipitated that use.
- Ask clients to write down their maladaptive thoughts on the handout.
- Discuss the group's examples.

Step 5: Brainstorm and discuss ways to manage maladaptive thoughts (approximately 15 minutes).

- Have group members remember times when they "let go" or "ignored" a thought that could have resulted in substance use.
- Discuss how they successfully did this and write these suggestions on the chalkboard/flipchart.
- Review ways to redirect thoughts and write them on chalkboard/flipchart.
- Discuss all the suggestions for managing thoughts.
- Ask clients to write any suggestions they feel would help in managing thoughts on the bottom of the handout.

Step 6: Close the session (approximately 5 minutes).

- Summarize the session and check in with group members.
- Ask group members to begin "noticing" their thoughts and to practice managing thoughts that could lead to substance use.

MALADAPTIVE THOUGHTS

Part I. Maladaptive Thoughts Sound Like This . . .

Write some examples of thoughts that can lead to substance use and get you into trouble.

Part II. Ways I Can Manage Maladaptive Thoughts

Write down some things you can do to stop the thought from leading to a harmful behavior.

Managing Cravings and Urges

CHANGE PROCESS OBJECTIVES: STIMULUS CONTROL, COUNTERCONDITIONING, REINFORCEMENT MANAGEMENT

RATIONALE

Like the previous session, this one combines the same three processes but, this time, in the service of learning to recognize and replace urges and cravings with healthier, more productive thoughts and behaviors. Clients can use *stimulus control* to alter tempting cues by *stopping* and redirecting a craving or urge before acting on it. They will be utilizing *counterconditioning* by *replacing* cravings and urges with healthy, substance-free thoughts and actions. Finally, the positive consequence of avoiding substance use will *reinforce* clients' efforts to manage cravings and urges in the future.

CONTENT OBJECTIVES

Clients discuss cravings and urges, and will be able to distinguish the difference between them.

Clients learn how to replace cravings and urges with positive thoughts and behaviors.

MATERIALS REQUIRED

Copies of the "To Manage Cravings and Urges I Can . . . " handout (A/M-9.1) for distribution to each group member

Pens and pencils

SESSION SUMMARY

The therapist facilitates a discussion regarding cravings and urges. The group discusses ways to manage cravings and urges, acknowledging the craving/urge, addressing unhealthy thoughts, changing the situation, and talking to someone. Clients write down specific examples of things they will do in the event that they experience a craving or an urge.

IMPLEMENTATION

Today's session focuses on cravings and urges. A *craving* can be seen as a desire to experience the positive effects of alcohol or drugs, whereas an *urge* can be thought of as an impulse to satisfy a craving (Marlatt & Gordon, 1985). It is important to note the difference between cravings–urges and maladaptive thoughts. Specifically, cravings–urges occur for only short periods, while maladaptive thoughts can actually strengthen and last a longer period of time. This session assists clients in understanding that unhealthy thoughts frequently occur simultaneously with cravings–urges and, as such, can make them much more difficult to address. As a result, one component of resisting cravings–urges involves addressing unhealthy thoughts as well.

(*Note.* As in the previous one, this session has the potential to be very rich in terms of content, although there are not as many activities as are found in other sessions. This is an especially relevant topic for clients who have stopped using alcohol and other drugs. Emphasize this by encouraging clients to share information from their experiences and engaging them in in-depth discussions.)

Steps 1 and 2: Open the Session and Introduce the Session Topic

Begin this session by pointing out the following:

- The key to understanding cravings and urges is that they are *time specific*. They are different from unhealthy thoughts, which can strengthen and last a significant amount of time.
- Because cravings and urges can seem quite powerful when they begin, it is crucial for clients to begin addressing them as soon as they realize what is happening; that is, because they only occur for a limited time, if they can be resisted, they will weaken and then disappear.
- Unhealthy thoughts frequently occur when a person has been exposed to a "trigger" situation. Explain that cravings and urges often occur "right behind" unhealthy thoughts. However, sometimes clients can have a craving or urge and *then* experience unhealthy thoughts as a result. In either case, unhealthy thoughts can cause cravings or urges to be more difficult to address.

Facilitate a group discussion regarding cravings and urges. Have the group members share their experiences with cravings and urges, and ask them what has and has not worked for them as they tried to resist cravings and urges.

Step 3: Discuss Ways to Manage Cravings and Urges

Distribute the "To Manage Cravings and Urges I Can . . . " handout (A/M-9.1). Emphasize that if clients are able to resist cravings and urges for the first few minutes, it is likely that they can successfully avoid using alcohol or other drugs. Explain that in doing so, it is helpful to begin by acknowledging when they are experiencing a craving or urge. One way to do this is to vocalize that they are having a craving–urge (as they learned to do in the previous session with unhealthy thoughts). For example, a client might say aloud, "I am really craving a drink right now."

Then, it is important for the client to address any maladaptive thoughts that may accompany the craving–urge. Clients can do so by asking themselves questions similar to those that they learned in the previous session (i.e., Could these thoughts "cause trouble"? and so on). Suggest that it can also be helpful to remember the pros of abstinence and the cons of drinking or drug use to help manage these thoughts. Remind clients of the previous sessions in which they discussed the "good things" and the "not so good things" about their substance use.

Another way to address maladaptive thoughts that occur with cravings–urges is to begin to think actively of something else. Have clients decide on three substance-free things that they will begin thinking of whenever they experience a craving or urge; these can be events, people, or even places that are special to them in some way. Examples could be the birth of a child, earning a raise or promotion at work, or simply a loved one. Ask them to write their own examples on their handout. (This activity encourages the change process of counterconditioning.)

Another useful tool in addressing unhealthy thoughts that occur with cravings or urges is simply to remember substance-related successes. Have clients think about small steps they have taken toward changing their substance use, or even goals that they have met in terms of their alcohol or drug use. Examples would be removing all of the drugs/alcohol from their home, reducing the amount that they have been using, or quitting altogether. Ask clients to write a few of their successes on their handouts. (*Note.* This activity encourages the change process of reinforcement management. If a client has difficulty in generating successes, suggest that being a member of this group, attending on a regular basis, and helping other group members during sessions are three important successes that they should not take for granted.)

Other helpful techniques to address cravings and urges include changing the situation and talking to another person about the craving–urge. Ask clients to write down three places they can go that might help the craving or urge subside. Examples might be going to church, taking a drive in a car, or even simply going for a walk outside. (This encourages the change process of stimulus control.) Also, have clients write the names or initials of two people that they can talk to whenever they being to have a craving or urge to drink or use other drugs. (*Note.* If clients are unable to think of support people, suggest that they write down your name and the name of another group member.)

Step 4: Close the Session

Summarize the session by reviewing information about cravings and urges and checking in with members to address any remaining issues. If group members have any other suggestions for effective ways to address cravings and urges, have them describe these and write them down on the handout as well. Emphasize that cravings and urges can be the most tempting events, and, as such, clients should utilize as many tools as possible to resist them.

STEP-BY-STEP SESSION TASKS

Step 1: Open the session and briefly check in with group members (approximately 10 minutes).

Step 2: Introduce the session topic: Managing cravings and urges (approximately 15 minutes).

- Facilitate group discussion involving members' experiences with cravings and urges (What works? What doesn't?).
- Discuss similarities–differences between cravings–urges and unhealthy thoughts.

Step 3: Discuss ways to manage cravings and urges (approximately 20 minutes).

- Distribute the "To Manage Cravings and Urges I Can..." handout (A/M-9.1).
- Explain the importance of acknowledging the craving–urge.
- Discuss ways to address maladaptive thoughts that might occur.
- Discuss options of changing or leaving the situation and talking to someone.
- Have clients write personal, specific examples on the handout.

Step 4: Close the session (approximately 10 minutes).

- Summarize the session and check in with group members.
- Have clients write down any additional ways to address cravings and urges.

TO MANAGE CRAVINGS AND URGES I CAN . . .

Acknowledge the craving or urge

State out loud that I am having a craving or urge to use alcohol or drugs.

Address maladaptive thoughts

1. Ask myself questions such as the following:

   - What thoughts am I having?
   - Could these thoughts "cause trouble"?
   - What expectations do I have about the alcohol or drug use?
   - Are these realistic expectations?
   - What are the possible consequences of this action?
   - If I were in a different mood, place, or time, would I be making the same decision?

2. Remember the "pros" of abstinence and the "cons" of drinking or drug use.
3. Think of something else. Things I can think of are as follows:

   _____   _____   _____

4. Encourage myself.
   - Remember all the successes I have had.
   - Remember how hard I have tried, and how far I have come.
   - Some of my successes are as follows:

   _____   _____   _____

Change the situation
   - I can leave the situation or do something else.
   - Places I can go are as follows:

   _____   _____   _____

Talk to someone
   - I can ask someone else for some support and help.
   - The people I can talk to are as follows:

   _____   _____   _____

New Ways to Enjoy Life

CHANGE PROCESS OBJECTIVES: STIMULUS CONTROL, COUNTERCONDITIONING, REINFORCEMENT MANAGEMENT

RATIONALE

This session helps clients to learn new, healthy behaviors to substitute for their previous activities that centered around alcohol and other drug use. Clients can use the change process of *stimulus control* to *avoid* engaging in activities are linked with alcohol and drug use. By *replacing* tempting activities with healthy, substance-free ones, clients will be using the change process of *counterconditioning*. Finally, the positive consequence of avoiding substance use will *reinforce* clients' efforts to participate in healthy substance-free activities in the future.

CONTENT OBJECTIVES

Clients identify alcohol- and drug-free activities that they can enjoy.
Clients identify potential problems in substituting new activities for less healthy ones.
Clients brainstorm solutions to those potential problems.

MATERIALS REQUIRED

Copies of "Alternatives to Using" handout (A/M-10.1) for distribution to each group member
Chalk and chalkboard or flipchart and markers
Pens or pencils

SESSION SUMMARY

Clients discuss whether they can continue to participate in some activities in which they previously engaged while they were using alcohol and/or drugs. The group brainstorms options for substance-free activities, possible roadblocks to these activities, and potential solutions to the roadblocks. The technique of brainstorming was introduced in earlier sessions in this manual.

IMPLEMENTATION

Many times, clients feel that they are "missing out" on a good time as a result of their abstinence; it's as if life isn't as much fun without alcohol or drugs. In fact, many people who have stopped using alcohol or other drugs describe their "new" lives as *boring*. There are simply "gaps" in their day, when they used to be busy engaging in substance-abusing activities. Healthy, enjoyable, substance-free activities the clients can substitute for the "old" activities that centered around alcohol or other drugs are needed. This will be addressed in today's session, and group members will brainstorm some suggestions of activities they can enjoy without using alcohol or drugs.

Steps 1 and 2: Open the Session and Introduce the Topic

After briefly checking in with the group, introduce the topic. Stress that it is important to learn new, enjoyable behaviors that can be substituted for their old activities (the majority of which most likely involved alcohol or other drug use). Mention that, oftentimes, people complain of boredom after they quit using because so much of their time was taken up by the substance abuse. Facilitate a discussion to help clients identify specific times during their day (or week) when boredom or restlessness (i.e., "I just don't know what to do with myself!") might set in. For some, this might be in the evening, or for others every Friday night—that is, times when they used to be occupied by their substance use activities.

Step 3: Generate Alternate Activities

Distribute the "Alternatives to Using" handout (A/M-10.1). Have group members brainstorm different alcohol- and drug-free activities they can enjoy. Ask for examples of things group members are currently doing that they enjoy, and discuss things they have done in the past as well. Write these suggestions on the chalkboard/flipchart as group members respond. Are there some activities that they used to do (while using alcohol/drugs) that could be just as fun without them? Suggestions might be spending time with friends, watching sports on television, and listening to music. Are there other activities they would like to try? Discuss this with the group, pointing out that for some clients, these activities might tempt them to use again, while for others, this can be a strong reinforcement that they no longer depend on substance abuse to fill their time.

Have the group write possible activities on the far left-hand column of the chart on the worksheet.

Step 4: Identify Potential Roadblocks

Have clients think about things that might "get in the way" of these activities. Choose a few suggestions from the chalkboard/flipchart to demonstrate examples of potential roadblocks. For example, a potential problem for someone who wanted to play sports might be a lack of equipment (tennis racket, basketball, and so on). Write these examples on the chalkboard/flipchart next to their respective activities. Have the clients write and discuss potential problems or distractions for the activities they have written on their handout.

Step 5: Problem-Solve the Roadblocks

Tell the group that it can often be helpful to try and solve potential problems or difficulties before they actually arise. Using the examples you have written on the chalkboard/flipchart, have clients discuss things that get in the way and ways to overcome those barriers; write these on the chalkboard/flipchart. Have clients think about the roadblocks they identified on their handouts. Have the group share these roadblocks; facilitate a group discussion of suggestions to address these potential problems. Have the clients write down several options for each potential problem.

Step 6: Close the Session

Briefly check in with the group members, then summarize the session by emphasizing that life does not have to be boring or dull simply because they no longer use alcohol or other drugs. Stress that it is "normal" to feel restless or bored at times, because they have been so used to engaging in substance abuse activities that there is a natural void when those activities disappear. Ask group members to begin adding the alternate activities to their daily routines. Encourage them to try at least one of the activities between now and the next session.

STEP-BY-STEP SESSION TASKS

Step 1: Open the session and check in with group members (approximately 5 minutes).

Step 2: Introduce the topic: New ways to enjoy life (approximately 10 minutes).

- Emphasize the importance of substituting new pleasurable activities for the old, unhealthy, substance-abusing behaviors.
- Point out that many people who have quit using complain of boredom or restlessness.

- Facilitate discussion to help clients identify particular times during the day when they may feel bored or restless.

Step 3: Generate alternate activities (approximately 10 minutes).

- Distribute the "Alternatives to Using" handout (A/M-10.1).
- Are there some activities clients used to do (while using alcohol/drugs) that could be just as fun without them?.
- Have the group brainstorm alcohol- and drug-free activities.
- Write examples on the chalkboard/flipchart.
- Have the group write possible activities on the far-left-hand column of the worksheet.

Step 4: Identify potential roadblocks (approximately 10 minutes).

- Have the group think about things that might get in the way of these activities.
- Choose a few activities and write these examples on the chalkboard/flipchart to demonstrate examples of roadblocks.
- Have clients write and discuss potential problems in doing the activities they have written on their handouts.

Step 5: Problem-solve the roadblocks (approximately 15 minutes).

- Point out that it can be helpful to try to solve potential problems before they occur.
- Use the examples on the chalkboard/flipchart to demonstrate how to generate possible solutions.
- Write these solutions on the chalkboard/flipchart.
- Ask group members to share their roadblocks and discuss possible solutions to address these problems.
- Have the group write down several options for each potential problem.

Step 6: Close the session (approximately 10 minutes).

- Briefly check in with group members.
- Summarize the session.
- Encourage group members to try at least one of the activities between now and the next session.

ALTERNATIVES TO USING

The following are some enjoyable activities that I can do without alcohol or other drugs, things that might get in the way, and possible solutions to those things:

Activity	Things That Might Get in the Way	Solutions

Developing an Action Plan

CHANGE PROCESS OBJECTIVE: SELF-LIBERATION

RATIONALE

Self-liberation involves belief in one's ability to change and acting on that belief by making a commitment to alter behavior. This session is designed to assist clients with acknowledging that they are capable of making effective changes in their lives by committing to an action plan using tools with which they are familiar.

CONTENT OBJECTIVES

Client review techniques to avoid using alcohol and other drugs.
Have clients choose which techniques work best for them personally.
Assist clients in writing out an action plan.

MATERIALS REQUIRED

Copies of the following for distribution to each group member:
   "Review" handout (A/M-11.1)
   "My Action Plan" handout (A/M-11.2)

SESSION SUMMARY

Facilitators review each of the topics and tools covered in the group thus far. Clients choose which techniques/tools are most useful for them in avoiding substance use and write these in detail in the form of an "action" plan.

IMPLEMENTATION

Today's session is devoted to helping clients actually write down a plan of action that best fits them personally by incorporating tools and techniques with which they feel most comfortable. This can be seen as a critical process in that clients will express their personal responsibility to stay abstinent and agree to abide by plans of their own creation. Also, recommend that clients ask important people in their lives to acknowledge this plan and support them as they attempt to remain alcohol- and drug-free.

Steps 1 and 2: Open the Session and Introduce the Topic

Briefly check in with group members and introduce the idea of creating an action plan. Point out that because everyone is unique, not all the techniques will be useful for every single person in the group. Tell clients that the purpose of today's session is to help them develop their own, individualized action plans, using the skills they have learned during the previous sessions.

Step 3: Review Techniques and Tools for Avoiding Substance Use

Distribute the "Review" handout (A/M-11.1). Explain that, to begin, you will be reviewing each of the topics and techniques you have introduced to the group. Read Part I completely, reviewing and summarizing the key points for each topic with the group members. Ask group members if they remember any further information for the topics that you may have "left out" of this summary.

Read Part II aloud, reviewing each technique as you do so. Facilitate a discussion with group members, asking them about their experiences in using these tools since the group began meeting. Have they been doing anything else to avoid using alcohol or other drugs that is not included on this list or covered in the group? If so, what? Have clients write any additional helpful tools at the end of the lists. Be sure to affirm clients for having tried to use the tools and techniques you have introduced during the group.

Step 4: Create an Action Plan

Ask the clients to write a check mark in the blanks beside the tools that they have found to be effective and helpful in avoiding alcohol and other drug use. Distribute the "My Action Plan" handout (A/M-11.2). Have the clients choose six of the tools that they checked as being the most useful in remaining alcohol- and drug-free. Ask the group to write these six tools on the "My Action Plan" handout, being as specific as possible. For instance, if the tool used is "Ask someone for help," the client should add names or descriptions of people whom he or she should contact, as well as where to find these people. The more specific the plans can be, the better. When a strong temptation to use arises, the more information the clients have available, the more it may help them to think clearly and not panic. By having several specific options, clients are more likely to use tools to avoid substance use.

Step 5: Close the Session

When everyone has completed the action plan, facilitate a group discussion. What are clients' concerns about the plans? Emphasize that they have been trying these tools and techniques throughout the course of the group. Affirm clients who, when faced with tempting situations, have resisted the urge to use. Stress that they *can* remain drug- and alcohol-free, and have demonstrated this by taking (in some cases) small steps and (in others) big ones. Summarize the session and highlight the importance of "sticking to" their personal commitments to remaining sober, and alcohol- and drug-free. Encourage group members to share their action plans with important people in their lives who can support and help them implement the plans.

STEP-BY-STEP SESSION TASKS

Step 1: Open the session and check in with the group members (approximately 10 minutes).

Step 2: Introduce the topic: Developing an action plan (approximately 10 minutes).

- Point out that not all techniques will be useful for all group members.
- Explain that, today, clients will develop an action plan that incorporates tools that are effective for them.

Step 3: Review techniques and tools for avoiding substance use (approximately 15 minutes).

- Distribute the "Review" handout (A/M-11.1).
- Read Part I aloud, reviewing and summarizing key points for each topic.
- Ask the group if you have left out any important information.
- Read Part II aloud, reviewing each technique.
- Facilitate a group discussion.
- Have clients write additional tools at the end of the list, if they wish.

Step 4: Create an action plan (approximately 15 minutes).

- Have the clients write a check mark in the blanks beside the tools they feel are the most effective for them.
- Distribute the "My Action Plan" handout (A/M-11.2).
- Ask the clients to choose six of the tools that they checked as being the most helpful and write them on the handout.
- Ask clients to personalize the techniques on their action plans by writing specific details.

Step 5: Close the session (approximately 10 minutes).

- Facilitate a group discussion regarding the plans.
- Recognize clients who have resisted temptations to use.
- Emphasize that group members have proven they can remain alcohol and drug-free by taking both small and large steps toward abstinence.
- Encourage the group members to share their action plans with important people in their lives.

REVIEW

Part I: In our group sessions we learned about:

Identifying triggers and planning to avoid or alter trigger situations
- When struggling with withdrawal?
- When having physical pain?
- When having negative feelings?
- When in social/positive situations?

Altering your response to triggers by managing maladaptive thoughts
- Pay attention to maladaptive thoughts (say out loud).
- Stop before acting on a thought.
- Think about consequences.
- Do something else.

Rewarding successes
- Acknowledge accomplishments.
- Reward steps toward maintaining change.

Giving Feedback
- Stay calm.
- Choose a right time/place.
- Correct misunderstandings.
- Don't blame.
- Use "I" language.

Altering your response to triggers by managing stress
- Pay attention to physical tension.
- Pay attention to emotional stress.
- Use relaxation techniques.

Managing cravings and urges
- Remember they are time-limited.
- Notice maladaptive thoughts.
- Wait an hour before using.
- Remember successes.
- Call someone for support.

Enjoying life
- It is normal to feel bored or restless.
- Do alcohol- and drug-free activities.

Assertiveness
- Describe the problem behavior.
- Describe your feelings or reactions.
- Describe what you want to see happen.

Effective refusals
- Pay attention to body language.
- Do not engage in argument.
- "No" is really enough.

Handling criticism/conflict
- Stay cool.
- Listen.
- Correct misunderstandings.

(continued)

Part II: Tools I Have Learned for Avoiding Substance Use

_____ Pay attention to "triggers"

_____ Think of possible consequences

_____ Delay the decision

_____ Change the situation

_____ Speak assertively

_____ Change activities

_____ Pay attention to your thoughts

_____ Remember the pros and cons

_____ Call someone—Ask for help

_____ Use relaxation techniques

_____ Reward successes

_____ "No" is enough

_____ Give feedback appropriately

_____ Handle receiving feedback

_____ Do substance-free activities

_____ Distract my thoughts

MY ACTION PLAN

I understand that even though I have stopped using alcohol and/or drugs, I will still be tempted to use.

I understand that having a "slip" does *not* mean that I am a failure. I will learn from that setback and try again. I agree to accept my responsibility and try to avoid relapsing.

I understand that I am not doing this alone, and that I have people in my life who can support me and help me stay away from alcohol and/or drugs.

If I start to feel tempted, I will . . .

1.

2.

3.

4.

5.

6.

Recommitting after a Slip

CHANGE PROCESS OBJECTIVE: SELF-LIBERATION

RATIONALE

Self-liberation involves belief in one's ability to change and acting on that belief by making a commitment to alter behavior. A slip or relapse is often a devastating occurrence in terms of self-concept and belief in ability to change. By reframing a slip as being a normal part of the cycle of change, clients are encouraged to learn from the experience and still see themselves in a positive light.

CONTENT OBJECTIVES

Clients understand that recycling through the stages of change is a normal part of behavior change.

Clients generate ideas for ways to recommit to changing substance use following a slip by beginning to move through the stages of change again.

MATERIALS REQUIRED

Copies of "What Can I Do after a Slip" handout (A/M-12.1) for distribution to each group member

SESSION SUMMARY

The facilitator explains that revisiting earlier stages of change is a normal part of behavior change and emphasizes that a slip does not mean a *failure*. Research shows that people often slip back into the problem behavior several times before changing successfully and maintaining the change. Clients discuss examples of times when they (or people they know) recycled through the stages of change when attempting to alter behavior. Based upon the stages of change, the group generates ideas for ways to "get back on track" and recommit to change following a slip.

IMPLEMENTATION

Unlike many traditional models, the stages of change model acknowledges that a "slip" or relapse is possible, even likely, during the process of behavior change. People often "recycle" through the stages many different times before successfully altering their behavior. Explain to clients that it took them a long time to learn all the behaviors related to their substance use, and it will also take a long time to "unlearn" those behaviors. Change takes a lot of time and energy, and we are not always successful the first time around; but each time a person attempts a change, he or she learns some important things about the behavior, for example, about the barriers to change and the areas in which he or she is most likely to encounter a slip. Clients can use this information in their subsequent attempts to change. This is often called "recycling" through the stages. During this recycling, people often return to an earlier stage and then begin progressing through the stages again. In this way, a slip should not be considered an utter failure but simply a temporary step back in the change process. You might also want to link this idea back to A/M Session 8, in which we discussed managing thoughts. Point out that if a person thinks of a slip as a total failure, it could become one, and he or she might give up and stop trying. By reframing a slip as a learning experience rather than as a failure, the potential for success increases.

Although many interventions address the issue of relapse only after it occurs, this manual takes a proactive approach by having clients prepare for a slip ahead of time. Remember that some group members may have experienced a slip in the past. By helping clients generate ideas about ways to recommit and "get back on track," you may be addressing an urgent need for some clients and anticipating that same need for others.

Steps 1 and 2: Open the Session and Introduce the Topic

Check in with group members and remind them that, unlike some other treatment programs, this intervention recognizes that a slip might occur on the way to changing behavior. A slip should be considered a normal part of the change process and *does not* mean failure. Explain that most people, when they are changing behavior, have a slip at one time or another and go back to an earlier stage of change.

Step 3: Discuss Examples of Recycling through the Stages of Change

Have clients think about a behavior that, though difficult to change, they were successfully able to do. Or they can think about someone they know who has made a significant behavior change that was not easy to do. Discuss these examples of change with the group, using questions such as the following:

- "Did the change come all at once, or did it take time to occur?"
- "Were there times when a slip happened?"
- "How did you 'get back on track'?"
- "After the slip, did you give up for a while, or did you start trying to change again right away?"

Give the following example to the group: A client named Bob had not smoked a cigarette for several months, and then he had a slip one weekend and smoked a few. Afterwards, he was not quite ready to stop smoking altogether again, but he did consider it by weighing the pros and cons, and removing the cigarettes from his house so that he would not smoke at home. In this case, it could be said that Bob moved back to the preparation stage of change after his slip. Again, emphasize that this is a *normal* part of behavior change. Facilitate a group discussion about this approach to slips. In what ways might one "get back on track" once a slip occurs?

Step 4: Identify What Was Helpful in the Past in Changing Substance Use

Explain to the group that following a slip, it can be beneficial to think about things that originally helped members to change their substance use. Point out that they have moved through the stages *at least once* before in order to get to where they were just before the slip. Facilitate a discussion using prompts such as the following:

- "In the past, what motivated you to start thinking about making changes in your substance use?"
- "What helped you begin to lean more toward changing your substance use?"
- "When did you decide to make small changes in your drinking or drug use?"
- "What helped you completely stop using alcohol and other drugs?"

Step 5: Discuss Ideas of Things to Do following a Slip

Distribute the "What Can I Do after a Slip?" handout (A/M-12.1). Explain that here are some suggestions of things to try after a slip has occurred. Read and discuss the suggestions on the handout for each of the stages of change.

Step 6: Close the Session

Briefly check in with the group and summarize the session by reminding clients that they are *not* failures if they have a slip. Emphasize to clients that it is a normal part of the change process to revisit an earlier stage of change following a slip, and that you have discussed ways to "get back on track" and recommit to changing their substance use in the event they do have a slip.

STEP-BY-STEP SESSION TASKS

Step 1: Open the session and check in with group members (approximately 5 minutes).

Step 2: Introduce the topic: Recommitting after a slip (approximately 10 minutes).

- Explain that a slip should be considered a normal part of the change process and *does not* mean failure.
- Point out that most people, when they are changing behavior, have a slip at one time or another and go back to an earlier stage of change.

Step 3: Discuss examples of recycling through the stages of change (approximately 10 minutes).

- Have clients think about a time when they (or someone they know) successfully changed a behavior.
- Using prompts, discuss whether they slipped and recycled through the stages in making this change.
- Give an example of how a person can recycle through the stages during the change process.
- Discuss this approach, emphasizing that recycling is a *normal* part of the change process.

Step 4: Identify what was helpful in the past in changing substance use (approximately 10 minutes).

- Explain that it can be beneficial to think about things that originally helped clients in changing their substance use.
- Facilitate a discussion using prompts.

Step 5: Discuss ideas of things to do following a slip (approximately 10 minutes).

- Distribute the "What Can I Do after a Slip?" handout (A/M-12.1).
- Explain that these are suggestions of things that clients can try following a slip, taking into account that they may now be in a different stage of change.
- Read and discuss the suggestions for each stage of change.

Step 6: Close the session (approximately 10 minutes).

- Check in with the group.
- Summarize the session.

WHAT CAN I DO AFTER A SLIP?

After a slip, you might find yourself in one of the following stages of change:

Precontemplation—You may be *doubting* that it's worth trying to change your substance use. If so, it may be helpful to do the following:

- Review information about how alcohol and other drugs can affect you physically, socially, or emotionally.
- Think about your values and whether using alcohol or other drugs conflicts with them.
- Think about how your substance use affects other people.

Contemplation—You may be *considering making changes* in your alcohol or drug use again, but you may not be quite sure. If so, it may be helpful to do the following:

- Think about the consequences for yourself of the behavior.
- Weigh the pros and cons.
- Think about what you expect to get out of using alcohol or other drugs, and if these are realistic expectations.

Preparation—You may decide that you want to *get ready to change* your alcohol or drug use again. If so, you might try the following:

- Take small steps toward behavior change.
- Start talking to people who have successfully quit using.
- Keep in mind the situations that led to the slip and think of ways to avoid them.
- Develop a change plan.

Action—You may decide that you *want to stop* using alcohol or drugs again. If so, then it will be helpful to do the following:

- Avoid or alter situations that tempt you to use.
- Change your responses to offers to use, stressful situations, and automatic thoughts.
- Reward yourself for successes.
- Interact with people who support your changes.
- Try to help others who are trying to quit.

A/M SESSION 13

Social Support

RATIONALE

Helping relationships are relationships that provide support, caring, and acceptance to someone who is attempting to make a change. This session will help clients identify their social support networks and become more aware of the current and potential helping relationships in their lives. It is also important for clients to acknowledge that it is their responsibility to ask for support. They should not wait for others to anticipate their needs. Clients are helped to realize the importance of being supportive to others.

CONTENT OBJECTIVES

Clients identify potential sources of social support.
Clients learn to develop further their social support networks.
Clients understand the importance of being a support to others.

MATERIALS NEEDED

Copies of "Where Do I Get Help?" handout (A/M-13.1) for distribution to each group member

SESSION SUMMARY

Facilitators assist clients in completing an exercise that identifies support networks and helping relationships via a diagram that includes numerous areas (e.g., medical, school, religion, friends, job, and so on). Clients also discuss ways that they can be supportive to others.

IMPLEMENTATION

Research has shown that healthy, supportive relationships are important in helping a person succeed in behavior change. Some clients may feel alone and not realize that they actually *do* have potential helping relationships. Today, you will help clients complete an exercise that is designed to identify potential and current support networks. You will assist group members in understanding that support is not a "one way street," and by being genuinely available to others, the support they receive will also increase. You will discuss ways clients can support and help others, in addition to reviewing assertiveness in asking for assistance.

Many people have grown up with the idea that asking for and accepting help is a sign of weakness. In order for this session to be successful, it will be important to address this issue. Remind clients that relationships are a fundamental part of being human. Much strength can be obtained through the healthy, positive aspects of relationships with others. This is especially valuable in trying to change alcohol and drug use. It will be important to take a few minutes to explore this issue with the group during the session.

Note that there may be clients in your group whose social support resources are lacking. In fact, it is likely that they have alienated friends and family members through years of substance abuse. You should help these clients brainstorm options for support and point out people that can usually be helpful (other group members, yourself, case managers, clergy, etc.). This is also a good opportunity to talk about the potential usefulness of Alcoholics Anonymous (AA) or other 12-step groups.

Steps 1 and 2: Open the Session and Introduce the Topic

After briefly checking in with group members, introduce the concept of helping relationships. Explain that helping relationships are important in making and maintaining behavior changes. Tell the group that you will be talking about the people who can support them during today's session. Stress that these relationship networks are frequently in place, but many people have difficulty in identifying them. So, today, group members will be completing an exercise to help them identify existing and potential helping relationships. Also, discuss the idea that asking for help is *not* a sign of weakness.

Explain to the group that the belief many people have grown up with is that it is shameful or "not okay" to ask for help. A more mature, practical way of looking at this is that it and will help clients to achieve their goals. While some people may feel that they can "go it alone," we maximize our chances for success when we include others as resources in our network of support.

Step 3: Identify Potential and Existing Supportive Relationships

Distribute the "Where Do I Get Help?" handout (A/M-13.1). Explain that clients will see several circles on the page, each representing areas that are sometimes a part of people's lives. Briefly review each of the areas aloud and point out some examples of people who can be supportive in each (such as nurse or case manager under the "Medical" circle).

Ask clients to think about the different places they go and the people they see every day. Have them write the names (or descriptions) of people who can help and encourage them in each circle. Explain that not everyone will use all of these areas, and in fact, there may be some group members with different categories that are not included on the sheet. If so, they can write the name of the category under one of the blank circles. Walk among the group, giving input and asking questions to help clients think of various sources of support. When everyone has finished, discuss this activity. Have different group members describe the types of people who help them (names are not necessary). Ask if was easy or hard to think of people who can be supportive. A variation of this exercise is to ask group members also to include people who are "just outside" the circle, with whom they would like to develop a closer relationship.

Point out to group members that they have a personal responsibility to seek support actively when they need it. Briefly review assertiveness skills, and ways of approaching and interacting with others.

Step 4: Identify Ways Clients Can Be Supportive

Stress to the group that just as it is helpful to have the support of other people, it is equally important to support others. Relating to others is *not a one-way street!* Have group members brainstorm and discuss ways that they can be supportive to other people. Have them think about specific people that they might be able to support or encourage. Ask if it is easier to identify people who support them or people whom they can support?

Step 5: Close the Session

Briefly check in with the group and summarize the session by reviewing the important role that healthy, supportive relationships play in maintaining behavior change. Encourage clients to thank those they identified today as supporters. These supporters may not even be aware of the help that they have given the clients. Also, ask group members to make a concerted effort to try and encourage or support three different people between now and the next session.

STEP-BY-STEP SESSION TASKS

Step 1: Open the session and check in with group members (approximately 5 minutes).

Step 2: Introduce the session topic: Social support (approximately 10 minutes).

- Explain that there is a basic human need for relationships.
- Explain that helping relationships are important in making behavior changes and are not a sign of weakness.
- Emphasize that social support networks are often in place, but sometimes it is hard to identify them.
- Discuss the fact that some people see asking for help as sign of weakness. Have clients examine their own feelings about whether this is true..

Step 3: Identify potential helping relationships (approximately 20 minutes).

- Distribute the "Where Do I Get Help?" handout (A/M-13.1).
- Review each of the areas, giving examples of people who can be supportive in each.
- Have clients write descriptions or names of people who can support them in each circle.
- Circulate, giving input, and ask probing questions.
- Discuss this activity.
- Briefly review assertiveness skills and ways of approaching and interacting with others.

Step 4: Identify ways clients can be supportive (approximately 15 minutes).

- Point out that relating to others is *not a one-way street*.
- Have clients brainstorm and discuss ways that they can be supportive to other people.
- Ask clients to think of specific people that they might be able to support or encourage.

Step 5: Close the session (approximately 10 minutes).

- Briefly check in with the group.
- Summarize the session.
- Ask clients to thank their supporters and to encourage or support three people between now and the next session.

WHERE DO I GET HELP?

Think about the different places you go and people you see every day. Describe or write the names of people who help and encourage you in each circle.

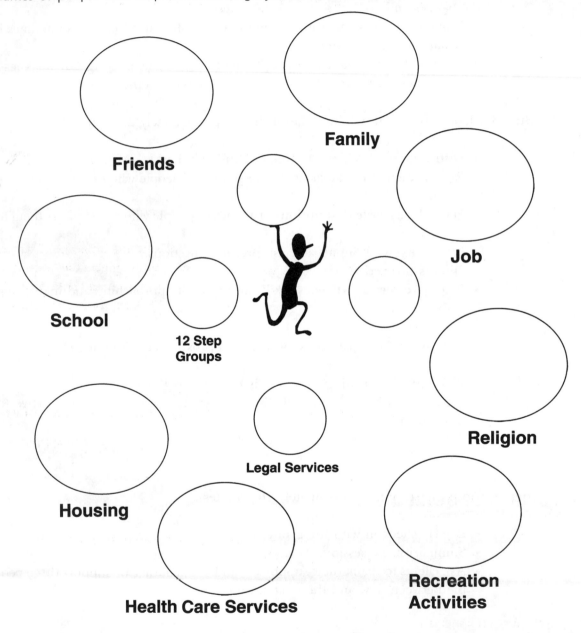

Identifying Needs and Resources

CHANGE PROCESS OBJECTIVE: SOCIAL LIBERATION

RATIONALE

Social liberation involves increasing alternatives for nonproblematic behavior. This session has clients identify areas of their lives that may have been neglected as a result of substance use and begin the process of locating resources to strengthen those areas. By addressing deficits in non-substance-related areas, clients will have the opportunity to live healthier, more balanced lives.

CONTENT OBJECTIVES

Clients identify areas of their lives that have not been fully developed as a result of alcohol or drug use.

Clients identify places to obtain information and assistance in developing these areas.

MATERIALS REQUIRED

Copies of the following handouts for distribution to each group member:
"Needs Assessment" handout (A/M-14.1)
"Resource Guide" handout (A/M-14.2)

SESSION SUMMARY

The facilitator explains that years of substance use can often result in clients' neglect of other areas of their lives. It is often helpful for clients to identify which areas they may have neglected. Clients complete a needs assessment in which they identify those areas that are currently "under control" and those that "could use improvement." The facilitator distributes a detailed chart that summarizes where to locate various resources and leads the group through an example of how to link a personal need with a resource that can facilitate meeting that need.

IMPLEMENTATION

Prior to clients' stopping their use, alcohol- and drug-related activities probably occupied a substantial portion of their time. If the substance use continued over many years, a great deal of their lives has most likely been spent in substance-related activities. Practically speaking, less time was available for nonusing activities, and other areas of their lives may have been ignored or neglected. Many times, clients need to strengthen the areas they may have neglected in order to function well and minimize the potential for future problems. They may have some "catching up" to do in order to meet their basic needs and to live healthy, well-rounded lives. This session helps clients to identify those areas that could use improvement and teaches them how to locate resources to strengthen those areas.

Steps 1 and 2: Open the Session and Introduce the Topic

Explain that there are basic needs common to every human. Although the way these needs are met may differ from person to person, and culture to culture, meeting these needs helps people live healthier and more satisfying lives. Point out that while they were using alcohol and/or other drugs, clients most likely neglected some other areas of their lives in which they have needs. Explain that they may have some "catching up to do" in order to meet their basic needs and live healthy, balanced lives.

Step 3: Identify Areas Needing Improvement

Distribute the "Needs Assessment" handout (A/M-14.1), explaining that it lists categories that represent basic needs common to every human. Read through each category and the corresponding examples. For each category, have clients determine whether they currently have that area "Under control" or whether that area "Needs improvement." Indicate this by placing a check mark in either of those columns. Note that there are additional spaces under the examples for each category so that clients can add any specific topic they feel they have under control or could improve.

When they have finished, tell clients that they have just identified some "strengths" and some "needs." Ask the group members to share what they noticed in completing this exercise. Point out that everyone is different. And some group members may have certain areas under control, while other clients may need to improve those areas. Emphasize that both the importance of each category and whether it is under control or could use some attention is really up to each group member, and that this may change from year to year.

Step 4: Practice Identifying Resources to Address Needs

Explain to the group that the next step in strengthening the "needs" that they have identified is to explore possible resources that could assist in improving them. Give the group an example of how to use resources to begin to meet a need. For example, a client defaulted on his college loans several years ago because of his substance use but would now like to go back to school. He has identified the area of "Education" as needing improvement, and he now needs to use resources to meet this need. He looks for information that can point him toward appropriate resources. In order to find this information, he decides to go to the Financial Aid Office at a local community college or university for consultation. They advise him as to what steps he has to take in order to resolve the problem, and he is able to reenroll the next semester.

Distribute the "Resource Guide" handout (A/M-14.2). Point out that although this is not a comprehensive list, it is a good starting point and may guide clients in the "right direction" to locate valuable resources. Ask clients to take a few minutes and choose one category on the "Needs Assessment" handout (A/M-14.1) that could use improvement. Then, have them find an organization that might be helpful on the "Resource Guide" handout (A/M-14.2) and write this next to the category on the "Needs Assessment" handout. Explain that this is how to identify resources that might help them address needs. You may wish to distribute a local resource guide at the end of this session.

Step 5: Close the Session

Briefly check in with the group and summarize the session by pointing out that although resources can be helpful in providing information and often assist with problem-solving situations, the ultimate responsibility to make improvements still lies within the clients themselves. Encourage clients to review the areas that they have marked as needing improvement during the next few months and to contact appropriate resources to begin addressing those needs.

STEP-BY-STEP SESSION TASKS

Step 1: Open the session and check in with group members (approximately 10 minutes).

Step 2: Introduce the topic: Identifying needs and resources (approximately 10 minutes).

- Explain that there are basic needs common to every human.
- Point out that while they were using substances, clients may have neglected other areas or needs in their lives.

Step 3: Identify areas needing improvement (approximately 15 minutes).

- Distribute the "Needs Assessment" handout (A/M-14.1).
- Read the categories aloud.
- Have clients mark whether each category is "Under control" or "Needs improvement."
- Have clients share what they learned in completing this exercise.
- Point out that everyone is different and that the importance or status of any given category for a person can change from year to year.

Step 4: Practice identifying resources to address needs (approximately 15 minutes).

- Give an example of how to use resources to begin to meet a need.
- Distribute the "Resource Guide" handout (A/M-14.2).
- Explain that although this is not a comprehensive list, it can point them in the right direction in locating resources.
- Have clients choose one category from the "Needs Assessment" handout (A/M-14.1) and find a resource that might help them improve on the "Resource Guide" handout (A/M-14.2).

Step 5: Close the session (approximately 10 minutes).

- Check in with the group.
- Summarize the session.
- Encourage clients to review the areas that they have determined need improvement during the next few months and to contact the appropriate resources to begin addressing those needs.

NEEDS ASSESSMENT

Category	Examples	Under control	Needs improvement
Body	Health Food/diet Personal appearance		
Play	Sports Hobbies		
Sociability	Friends Coworkers Establishing trust with others		
Family	Marriage Having children Caring for elders		
Work	Job skills Particular responsibilities at your job		
Education	Literacy/GED College Learning competence in some area		
Career	Choosing a direction Preparing to participate in a profession Promoting yourself within a profession		
Money	Wages and salaries Budget Savings		
World	Politics Environment Social justice		
Dignity	Self-respect Self-esteem Standards of performance		
Situation	Temperament Moods General assessment of "how things are going"		
Spirituality	Religion Philosophy		

RESOURCE GUIDE

This guide contains some of the areas that you might need to strengthen and specific resources that can help you improve those areas. If you know the exact name of these organizations, you can locate their phone number or address by calling Directory Assistance or looking in the Business Section of a telephone directory. If you do not know the organization's exact name, you can use the Yellow Pages to look up the general category.

A few resources available in each city to find general information and assistance are as follows:

- The United Way organization
- Information desk at your local public library
- Your clergy
- The Internet

Area	Subcategory	Resources
Body	Physical	City or county health clinics Medical schools
	Mental	Psychiatry departments at medical schools Local Mental Health Association Family Service Centers Psychology Departments or clinics at local universities Crisis hotline Local branch of the State Mental Health Agency
	Substance abuse	Local Council on Alcohol and Drugs Substance abuse treatment programs at medical schools Alcoholics Anonymous, Narcotics Anonymous, Al-Anon, and so on
	Dental	City or county health clinics University dental schools
	Vision	University optometry schools
Education	Literacy/GED	Community colleges
	Student loans	Financial Aid office at community colleges or universities
	Career guidance	University testing office (may have a fee) Books at your local library
	General information	Admissions Office at community colleges or universities

Area	Subcategory	Resources
Work	Job training	Local branch of State Workforce Commission Community colleges Technical schools
	Job leads	Local branch of State Workforce Commission
Family	Marital or family counseling	Local Mental Health Association Family Service Associations or Centers Pastoral counseling through your church
	Child counseling	United Way Helpline Local Mental Health Association Family Service Associations or Center School counselor or social worker (for referrals)
	Domestic violence; Child abuse, neglect or sexual abuse	Family Service Associations or Centers Local Mental Health Association Local area Women's Shelter Police Department United Way Helpline Crisis hotline City or county Child Protective Services
Money	Budget/debt	Consumer Credit Counseling
	Public transportation	Local Workforce Commission (*may* be able to provide temporarily)
	Utilities assistance	United Way Helpline
Play	Organized sports or area parks and swimming pools	City Parks Department YWCA or YMCA Work- or church-sponsored activities Children's museums

Review and Termination

RATIONALE

In this session, clients think back over the course of the group and discuss the progress they have made toward behavior change.

CONTENT OBJECTIVES

Clients review the topics covered during the course of the group.
Clients discuss changes and progress group members have made.
Clients engage in termination activities.

MATERIALS REQUIRED

Note cards that you have prepared in advance for each client that list several accomplishments or successes that they have made during the course of the group.
Copies of the following for distribution to each group member:
"Review" handout (A/M-15.1)
Chalkboard/flipchart

SESSION SUMMARY

Clients review the topics covered in the previous sessions. The facilitator assists with termination by leading a discussion of how the group has affected the clients, what they expect in the coming weeks without the group, and potential barriers to maintaining their behavior change. The facilitator shares a few accomplishments/successes for each group member and then gives clients note cards on which these accomplishments/successes are written.

IMPLEMENTATION

Many people have difficulty ending relationships in a healthy way, and a therapeutic setting provides an opportunity to practice this skill. In today's session, you will help group members do this by summarizing their experiences during the group. You will also review each of the major topics covered during the group sessions.

Steps 1 and 2: Open the Session and Introduce the Topic

Begin by briefly checking in with the group. Introduce the topic by explaining that, because this is the final session, you will be reviewing all of the topics covered throughout the course of the group. Point out that you will be helping the clients to summarize their experiences during the group.

Step 3: Review the Group Topics

Explain that because you have covered so much information throughout the course of the group, it will be helpful to review the topics. Distribute the "Review" handout (A/M-15.1). Read the topics and respective questions aloud, discussing each with the clients. Ask clients how their answers differ now from when you first discussed the subject.

Step 4: Conduct a Staging Exercise

Point out that, as a facilitator, you have been paying attention to how the clients have progressed during the course of the group. Ask them to think about whether they feel they have moved forward or stayed "about the same" in terms of their alcohol/drug use, answering only to themselves. On a chalkboard/flipchart, draw the stages of change diagram (see A/M Session 1) or distribute the "Stages of Change" handout (AM-1.1), and briefly summarize each stage. Ask the clients to look at each stage as you describe it and determine their own current stage. Discuss this restaging with the group. Is their stage different now than it was earlier in the group?

Step 5: Facilitate Termination Process

Point out that this group has most likely been a source of support to its members for quite some time and that clients should not feel "abandoned" simply because they will no longer meet as a group on a regular basis. Remind clients that they have all identified supporters who are present in their lives, and that perhaps now some of the other group members have been added to that list. [This would be an appropriate place to provide the telephone number of a local crisis hotline or to review clients' options in the event of a substance use emergency (such as contacting your staff, if appropriate; going to the Emergency Room at local hospital; and so on.)]

Explain to clients that a helpful way to close a treatment group is to think back along the course of the group and see how the group has affected their lives. Facilitate a group discussion about this particular group, choosing two or three questions from the following list (model appropriate termination skills by being the first to answer):

- "Name two things you have learned in the group."
- "How has the group affected your life?"
- "Name one positive thing about at least one other group member."
- "What will be different for you without the group?"
- "What are some barriers that might prevent you from maintaining the changes you have made?"
- "Anything else you would like to say?"

Step 6: Close the Session

Summarize the session, then read the note cards you have prepared for each client (see "Materials Required" for further information). Give the note card to each client after you read it, so that he or she can take it home as a reminder of his or her progress. If you feel that it is appropriate, encourage group members to clap or otherwise congratulate each other as you read the cards. Check in with the clients one last time to close the group.

STEP-BY-STEP SESSION TASKS

Step 1: Open the session and check in with the group (approximately 5 minutes).

Step 2: Introduce the topic: Review and termination (approximately 5 minutes).

- Explain that because this is the final group, you will review all of the topic covered in the course of the group.
- Point out that you will be helping the clients to summarize their experiences during the group (i.e., help with termination).

Step 3: Review the group topics (approximately 15 minutes).

- Distribute the "Review" handout (A/M-15.1).
- Read several of the topics and their respective questions aloud.
- Discuss these with the clients.
- Ask the clients how their answers differ now from when you first discussed the subject.

Step 4: Conduct a staging exercise (approximately 10 minutes).

- Ask the clients to think about whether they have moved forward or stayed "about the same" regarding their alcohol/drug use during the group; have them answer only to themselves.
- Draw the stages of change diagram on a chalkboard/flipchart.
- Summarize each of the stages and have clients determine their current stage.
- Discuss this activity with the group.

Step 5: Facilitate the termination process (approximately 15 minutes).

- Emphasize that clients should not feel abandoned with the close of the group, since they still have their supporters.
- Point out that the clients have all identified supporters in their lives, and that some of the group members may have been added to that list.
- Review a local crisis hotline telephone number or explain the options clients have in the event of an emergency.
- Facilitate a discussion regarding how clients feel the group has affected their lives (be the first one to do this).

Step 6: Close the session (approximately 10 minutes).

- Summarize the session.
- Read each of the note cards that you have prepared (see "Materials Required").
- Give the note card to each member after you read it, so that he or she can take it as a reminder of his or her progress.
- Check in with the group.

REVIEW

Listed below are the topics we have covered in the course of this group. Each topic has one or two questions to help you remember specific information and to see if your answers are different now from when the group began.

- The Stages of Change—What are the five stages?

- Identifying "Triggers"—What are some situations in which people are most tempted to use?

- Managing Stress—How can you effectively handle stressful situations?

- Rewarding My Successes—Why is reinforcing your successes important?

- Effective Communication—What are the three styles of effective communication? Which is most effective?

- Effective Refusals—Since learning refusal skills, has there been a time that you have effectively refused an offer to use drugs or alcohol?

- Managing Criticism—What are some effective ways to give feedback, yet keep a positive relationship with another person?

- Managing Thoughts—Describe some ways you have learned to manage maladaptive thoughts that could lead to substance use.

- Managing Cravings and Urges—How do you deal with cravings and urges?

- New Ways to Enjoy Life—What new, pleasurable activities have you engaged in since this group began?

- Developing an Action Plan—In what ways has the action plan you developed been helpful? Have you had to revise your plan since you first developed it?

- Recommitting after a Slip—What would you recommend a person do after they experience a slip?

- Social Support—Who have you found who is supportive of you while you have been trying to change your substance use?

- Identifying Needs and Resources—Name one area in which you have taken steps to improve.

Professional Contacts
and Suggested Resources

REFERENCES

The following texts provide supplemental information that you might find helpful.

Center for Substance Abuse Treatment. (1999). Enhancing motivation for change in substance abuse treatment (DHHS Publication No. SMA 99-3354). Washington, DC: U.S. Government Printing Office.

Connors, G. J., Donovan, D. M., & DiClemente, C. C. (2001). *Substance abuse treatment and the stages of change.* New York: Guilford Press.

Ingersoll, K. A., Wagner, C. C., & Gharib, S. (2000). *Motivational groups for community substance abuse programs.* Richmond, VA: Mid-Atlantic Addiction Technology Transfer Center, Virginia Commonwealth University.

Kadden, R., Carroll, K., Donovan, D., Cooney, N., Monti, P., Abrams, D., Litt, M., & Hester, R. (1995). *Cognitive-behavioral coping skills therapy manual: A clinical research guide for therapists treating individuals with alcohol abuse and dependence* (Project MATCH Monograph Series, Vol. 3; NIH Publication No. 94-3724). Rockville, MD: National Institute on Alcohol Abuse and Alcoholism.

Marlatt, G. A, & Gordon, J. R. (Eds.). (1985). *Relapse prevention: Maintenance strategies in the treatment of addictive behaviors.* New York: Guilford Press.

Miller, W. R., & Rollnick, S. (1991). *Motivational interviewing: Preparing people to change addictive behavior.* New York: Guilford Press.

Miller, W. R., Zweben, A., DiClemente, C. C., & Rychtarik, R. G. (1995). *Motivational enhancement therapy manual.* Rockville, MD: National Institute on Alcohol Abuse and Alcoholism.

Monti, P. M., Abrams, D. B., Kadden, R. M., & Cooney, N. L. (1989). *Treating alcohol dependence: A coping skills training guide.* New York: Guilford Press.

Nowinski, J., Baker, S., & Carroll, K., (1995). *Twelve step facilitation therapy manual.* Rockville, MD: National Institute on Alcohol Abuse and Alcoholism.

Prochaska, J. O., Norcross, J. C., & DiClemente, C. C. (1994). *Changing for good.* New York: Avon Books.

Zackon, F., McAuliffe, W. E., & Ch'ien, J. M. N. (1993). *Recovery training and self-help.* Rockville, MD: National Institute on Drug Abuse.

FOR INFORMATION ON TRAINING

Motivational Interviewing Network of Trainers Website (list of trainers by state)
www.motivationalinterview.org

William R. Miller, PhD
Center on Alcoholism, Substance Abuse, and Addictions (CAASA)
University of New Mexico
2350 Alamo SE
Albuquerque, NM 87106
(505) 768-0139
wrmiller@unm.edu   *http://casaa.unm.edu*

Carlo C. DiClemente, PhD
University of Maryland Baltimore County
5401 Wilkens Avenue
Baltimore, MD 21228-5398
(410) 455-2415
diclemen@research.umbc.edu

Mary Marden Velasquez, PhD
Department of Family Practice and Community Medicine
University of Texas–Houston Medical School
6341 Fannin, Suite JJL.324
Houston, TX 77030-1501
(713) 500-7590
mvelasquez@uth.tmc.edu

Kathleen Carroll, PhD
Substance Abuse Center, Yale University School of Medicine
VA CT Healthcare Center (151D)
West Haven, CT 06516
(203) 937-34886 x7403
kathleen.carroll@yale.edu

HELPFUL WEBSITES

Motivational Interviewing Network of Trainers Website *http://www.motivationalinterview.org*

National Institute on Alcohol Abuse and Alcoholism
http://www.niaaa.nih.gov

National Institute on Drug Abuse
http://www.nida.nih.gov

Cancer Prevention Research Center
http://www.uri.edu/research/cprc   *http://motivation.interview.org*

References

American Psychiatric Association. (1994). *Diagnostic and statistical manual of mental disorders* (4th ed.). Washington, DC: Author.

Babor, T. F., de la Fuente, J. R., Saunders, J., & Grant, M. (1992). *The Alcohol Use Disorders Identification Test: Guidelines for use in primary health care*. Geneva, Switzerland: World Health Organization.

Bandura, A. (1986). The explanatory and predictive scope of self-efficacy theory. *Journal of Social and Clinical Psychology, 4*(3), 359–373.

Benson, H. (1975). *The relaxation response*. New York: Morrow.

Bertcher, H. J. (1993). *Group participation: Techniques for leaders and members*. Beverly Hills, CA: Sage.

Bigelow, G. E., Brooner, R. K., & Silverman, K. (1998). Competing motivations: Drug reinforcement vs. non-drug reinforcement. *Journal of Psychopharmacology, 12*(1), 8–14.

Botvin, G., & Wills, T. A. (1985). Personal and social skills training: Cognitive-behavioral approaches to substance abuse prevention. *National Institute on Drug Abuse: RMS, 63*, 8–49.

Brown, S. A., Goldman, M. S., Inn, A., & Anderson, L. R. (1980). Expectations of reinforcement from alcohol: Their domain and relation to drinking patterns. *Journal of Consulting and Clinical Psychology, 48*, 419–426.

Carbonari, J. P., & DiClemente, C. C. (2000). Using the transtheoretical model profiles to differentiate levels of alcohol abstinence success. *Journal of Consulting and Clinical Psychology, 68*(5), 810–817.

Carroll, K. (1998). *A cognitive-behavioral approach: Treating cocaine addiction* (NIDA Therapy Manuals for Drug Addiction, Manual 1, NIH Publication No. 98-4308). Rockville, MD: National Institute on Drug Abuse.

Collins, C., Kohler, C., DiClemente, R., & Wang, M. Q. (1999). Evaluation of the exposure effects of a theory-based street outreach HIV intervention on African-American drug users. *Evaluation and Program Planning, 22*(3), 279–293.

Connors, G. J., Donovan, D. M., & DiClemente, C. C. (2001). *Substance abuse treatment and the stages of change*. New York: Guilford Press.

Connors, G. J., O'Farrell, P. J., Cutter, H. S. G., & Thompson, D. L. (1987). Dose-related effects of alcohol among male alcoholics, problem drinkers, and non-problem drinkers. *Journal of Studies on Alcohol, 48*(5), 461–466.

DiClemente, C. (1991). Stages of Change and Motivational Interviewing. In W. R. Miller & S. Rollnick (Eds.), *Motivational interviewing: Preparing people to change addictive behavior.* New York: Guilford Press.

DiClemente, C. C., Carbonari, J. P., Montgomery, R. P. G., & Hughes, S. O. (1994). The Alcohol Abstinence Self-Efficacy Scale. *Journal of Studies on Alcohol, 55,* 141–148.

DiClemente, C. C., Fairhurst, S. K., & Piotrowski, N. A. (1995). The role of self-efficacy in the addictive behaviors. In J. Maddux (Ed.), *Self-efficacy, adaptation, and adjustment: Theory, research and application* (pp. 109–141). New York: Plenum Press.

DiClemente, C. C., & Prochaska, J. O. (1998). Toward a comprehensive, transtheoretical model of change. In W. Miller & N. Heather (Eds.), *Treating addictive behaviors* (pp. 3–24). New York: Plenum Press.

Flores, F. (1983). *Conversations for action.* Workshop, San Francisco, CA.

Flores, F., & Graves, M. (1986). *Permanent domains of concern.* Unpublished manuscript, Business Design Associates, Alameda, CA.

Friedman, A. S., & Utada, A. T. (1992). Effects of two group interaction models on substance-abusing adjudicated adolescent males. *Journal of Community Psychology,* 106–117.

Grimely, D. M., Prochaska, G. E., & Prochaska, J. O. (1997). Condom use adoption and continuation: A transtheoretical approach. *Health Education Research, 12*(1), 61–75.

Hester, R. K. (1995). Behavioral self-control training. In R. Hester & W. Miller (Eds.), *Handbook of alcoholism treatment approaches: Effective alternatives* (pp. 148–159). Boston: Allyn & Bacon.

Higgins, S. T. (1999). Potential contributions of the community reinforcement approach and contingency management to broadening the base of substance abuse treatment. In J. M. Tucker & D. M. Donovan (Eds.), *Changing addictive behavior: Bridging clinical and public health strategies* (pp. 283–306). New York: Guilford Press.

Higgins, S. T., & Silverman, K. (Eds.). (1999). *Motivating behavior change among illicit-drug abusers: Research on contingency management interventions.* Washington, DC: American Psychological Association.

Huszti, H. C. (1997). *Strategies for communicating with providers.* Centers for Disease Control and Macro International, Atlanta, GA.

Ingersoll, K. A., Wagner, C. C., & Gharib, S. (2000). *Motivational groups for community substance abuse programs.* Richmond, VA: Mid-Atlantic Addiction Technology Transfer Center, Virginia Commonwealth University.

Janis, F. L., & Mann, L. (1977). *Decisional making: A psychological analysis of conflict, choice, and commitment.* New York: Free Press.

Kabat-Zinn, J. (1990). *Full catastrophe living.* New York: Delacorte Press.

Kadden, R., Carroll, K., Donovan, D., Cooney, N., Monti, P., Abrams, D., Litt, M., & Hester, R. (1995). *Cognitive behavioral coping skills manual: A clinical research guide for therapists treating individuals with alcohol abuse and dependence* (Project MATCH Monograph Series, Vol. 3; NIH Publication No. 94-3724). Rockville, MD: National Institute on Alcohol Abuse and Alcoholism.

Kominars, K. D. (1997). A study of visualization and addiction treatment. *Journal of Substance Abuse Treatment, 14*(3), 213–223.

Malow, R. M., West, J. A., Corrigan, S. A., Pena, J. M., & Cunningham, S. C. (1994). Outcome of psychoeducation for HIV risk reduction. *AIDS Education and Prevention, 6*(2), 113–125.

Marcus, B. H., Pinto, B. M., Simkin, L. R., Audrain, J. E., & Taylor, E. R. (1994). Application of theoretical models to exercise behavior among employed women. *American Journal of Health Promotion, 9*(1), 49–55.

Marlatt, G. A., & Gordon, J. R. (Eds.). (1985). *Relapse prevention: Maintenance strategies in the treatment of addictive behaviors.* New York: Guilford Press.

McConnaughy, E. A., DiClemente, C. C., Prochaska, J. O., & Velicer, W. F. (1989). Stages of change in psychotherapy: A follow-up report. *Psychotherapy, 26,* 494–503.

McMurran, M. (1996). Alcohol, drugs and criminal behaviour. In C. Hollin (Ed.), *Working with offenders: Psychological practice in offender rehabilitation* (pp. 211–242). Chicester, UK: Wiley.

Miller, W. R. (1985). Motivation for treatment: A review with special emphasis on alcoholism. *Psychological Bulletin, 98*(1), 84–107.

Miller, W. R. (1987). Techniques to modify hazardous drinking patterns. In M. Galanter & H. Begletier (Eds.), *Recent developments in alcoholism* (Vol. 5, pp. 425–438). New York: Plenum Press.

Miller, W. R. (1989). Increasing motivation for change. In R. Hester & W. Miller (Eds.), *Handbook of alcoholism treatment approaches: Effective alternatives* (pp. 67–80). Boston: Allyn & Bacon.

Miller, W. R., Benefield, R. G., & Tonigan, J. S. (1993). Enhancing motivation for change in problem drinking: A controlled comparison of two therapist styles. *Journal of Consulting and Clinical Psychology, 61,* 455–461.

Miller, W. R., & Rollnick, S. (1991). *Motivational interviewing: Preparing people to change addictive behavior.* New York: Guilford Press.

Miller, W. R., Zweben, A., DiClemente, C. C., & Rychtarik, R. G. (1994). *Motivational enhancement therapy manual: A clinical research guide for therapists treating individuals with alcohol abuse and dependence* (Project MATCH Monograph Series, Vol. 2; NIH Publication No. 94-3723). Rockville, MD: National Institute on Alcohol Abuse and Alcoholism.

Monti, P. M., Abrams, D. B., Kadden, R. M., & Cooney, N. L. (1989). *Treating alcohol dependence: A coping skills training guide.* New York: Guilford Press.

Monti, P. M., & O'Leary, T. A. (1999). Coping and social skills training for alcohol and cocaine dependence. *Psychiatric Clinics of North America, 22*(2), 447–470.

National Institute on Alcoholism and Alcohol Abuse. (1999). *What you don't know can harm you* (NIH Publication No. 99-4323). Washington, DC: U.S. Government Printing Office.

Noonan, W. C., & Moyers, T. B. (1997). Motivational interviewing. *Journal of Substance Misuse, 2,* 8–16.

Pallonen, U. E., Leskinen, L., Prochasks, J. O., Willey, C. J., Kaariainen, R., & Salonen, J. T. (1994). A 20-year self-help smoking cessation manual intervention among middle-aged Finnish men: An application of the transtheoretical model. *Preventive Medicine, 23*(4), 507–541.

Perz, C. A., DiClemente, C. C., & Carbonari, J. P. (1996). Doing the right thing at the right time? The intersection of stages and processes of change in successful smoking cessation. *Health Psychology, 15,* 462–468.

Prochaska, J. O., & DiClemente, C. C. (1984). *The transtheoretical approach: Crossing traditional boundaries of treatment.* Homewood, IL: Dow Jones-Irwin.

Prochaska, J. O., DiClemente, C. C., & Norcross, J. C. (1992). In search of how people change: Applications to addictive behavior. *American Psychologist, 47,* 1102–1114.

Prochaska, J. O., Norcross, J. C., & DiClemente, C. C. (1994). *Changing for good.* New York: Avon Books.

Prochaska, J. O., Velicer, W. F., Rossi, J. S., Goldstein, M. G., Marcus, B., Rakowski, W., Fiore, C., Harlow, L. L., Redding, C. A., Rosenbloom, D., & Rossi, S. R. (1994). Stages of change and decisional balance for 12 problem behaviors. *Health Psychology, 13,* 39–46.

Project MATCH Research Group. (1997). Matching alcoholism treatments to client heterogeneity: Project MATCH post-treatment drinking outcomes. *Journal of Studies on Alcohol, 58,* 7–29.

Rakowski, W., Ehrich, B., Goldstein, M. G., Rimer, B. K., Pearlman, D. N., Clark, M. A., Velicer, W. F., & Woolverton, H. (1998). Increasing mammography among women aged 40–74 by use of a stage-matched tailored intervention. *Preventive Medicine: An International Devoted to Practice and Theory, 27*(5, Pt. 1), 748–756.

Rohrbach, L. A., Graham, J. W., Hansen, W. B., & Flay, B. R. (1987). Evaluation of resistance skills training using multitrait–mulitmethod role play skill assessments. *Health Education Research, 2*(4), 401–407.

Rollnick, S., Mason, P., & Butler, C. (1999). *Health behavior change: A guide for practitioners.* Edinburgh, Scotland: Churchill Livingstone.

Rohsenow, D. (1983). Drinking habits and expectancies about alcohol's effects for self versus others. *Journal of Consulting and Clinical Psychology, 51*(5), 752–756.

Sobell, L. C., & Sobell, M. B. (1992). Timeline follow-back: A technique for assessing self-reported ethonal consumption. In J. Allen & R. L. Litten (Eds.), *Measuring alcohol consumption: Psychosocial and biological methods* (pp. 41–72). Totowa, NJ: Humana Press.

Sobell, L. C., Cunningham, J. A., Sobell, M. B., Agrawal, S., Gavin, D. R., Leo, G. I., & Singh, K. N. (1996). Fostering self-change among problem drinkers: A proactive community intervention. *Addictive Behaviors, 21*, 817–833.

Stotts, A. L., DiClemente, C. C., Carbonari, J. P., & Mullen, P. D. (1996). Pregnancy and smoking cessation: A case of mistaken identity. *Addictive Behaviors, 21*(3), 1–13.

Stotts, A., DiClemente, C. C., & Mullen, P. (in press). *One-to-one: A motivational interviewing intervention for resistant smokers.* Manuscript under review.

Velasquez, M. M., Carbonari, J. P., & DiClemente, C. C. (1999). Psychiatric severity and behavior change in alcoholism: The relation of the transtheoretical model variables to psychiatric distress in dually diagnosed patients. *Addictive Behaviors, 24*(4), 481–496.

Velasquez, M. M., Crouch, C., vonSternberg, K., & Grosdanis, I. (2001). Motivation for change and psychological distress in homeless substance abusers. *Journal of Substance Abuse Treatment.*

Velicer, W. F., DiClemente, C. C., Prochaska, J. O., & Brandenburg, N. (1985). A decisional balance measure for assessing and predicting stage status. *Journal of Personality and Social Psychology, 56*, 1279–1289.

Velicer, W. F., & Prochaska, J. O. (1999). An expert system intervention for smoking cessation. *Patient Education and Counseling, 36*(2), 119–129.

Werch, C. E., Pappas, D. M., Carlson, J. M., & DiClemente, C. C. (1999). Six-month outcomes of an alcohol prevention program for inner-city youth. *American Journal of Health Promotion, 13*(4), 237–240.

Wing, D. M. (1991). Goal setting and recovery from alcoholism. *Archives of Psychiatric Nursing, 5*(3), 178–184.

Yalom, I. D. (1995). *The theory and practice of group psychotherapy* (4th ed.). New York: Basic Books.

Index

A/M sessions, 3
  1 stages of change model, 127
    consciousness raising (change process
      objective), 127
    handout/Stages of Change, 129–130, 133f
    handout/Where Am I?, 130, 134f
    implementation, 128
    session steps, 128–131
    session summary, 128
    session tasks, 131–132
  2 environmental restructuring, 12
    handout/When Am I the Most Tempted to
      Use?, 136, 139
    implementation, 136
    session steps, 136–137
    session summary, 135
    session tasks, 137
    stimulus control (change process objective),
      135
  3 relaxation, 12
    counterconditioning (change process
      objective), 140
    handout; Meditation, 142, 145
    implementation, 141
    session steps, 141–142
    session summary, 141
    session tasks, 142–144
  4 reinforcement, 12
    handout/Rewarding My Success, 148, 150
    implementation, 147
    reinforcement management (change process
      objective), 146
    session steps, 147–148
    session summary, 146–147
    session tasks, 148–149

  5 reinforcement, 12
    counterconditioning and reinforcement
      management (change process objectives),
      151
    handout/Effective Communication, 153,
      155
    implementation, 152
    session steps, 153–154
    session summary, 152
    session tasks, 154
  6 role plays, 12, 158
    counterconditioning and reinforcement
      management (change process objectives),
      156
    implementation, 157
    session handout/Practicing Refusals, 158,
      160
    session steps, 157–158
    session summary, 157
    session tasks, 159
  7 reinforcement, 12
    counterconditioning and reinforcement
      management (change process objectives),
      161
    handout/Managing Criticism, 162, 165
    implementation, 162
    session steps, 162–163
    session summary, 162
    session tasks, 163–164
  8 cognitive restructuring, 12
    handout/Maladaptive Thoughts, 168, 171
    implementation, 167, 190
    session steps, 167–169
    session summary, 167
    session tasks, 169–170

A/M sessions, 8 cognitive restructuring, (*cont.*)
    stimulus control, counterconditoning, and
        reinforcement management (change
        process objectives), 166
    9 cognitive restructuring, 12
        handout/To Manage Cravings and Urges I
            Can . . ., 174, 176
        implementation, 173
        session steps, 173–175
        session summary, 173
        session tasks, 175
        stimulus control, counterconditioning, and
            reinforcement management (change
            process objectives), 172
    10 cognitive restructuring, 12
        handout/Alternatives to Using, 178–179,
            181
        implementation, 178
        session steps, 178–179
        session summary, 178
        session tasks, 179–180
        stimulus control, counterconditioning, and
            reinforcement management (change pro-
            cess objectives), 177
    11 relapse prevention planning, 12
        handout/My Action Plan, 183, 188
        handout/Review, 183, 186–187
        implementation, 183
        self-liberation (change process objective),
            182
        session steps, 183–184
        session summary, 182
        session tasks, 184–185
    12 framing, 12
        handout/What Can I Do After a Slip?,
            191, 193
        implementation, 190
        self-liberation (change process objective), 189
        session steps, 190–191
        session summary, 189–190
        session tasks, 192
    13 social and communications skills
        enhancement, 13
        handout/Where Do I Get Help?, 196, 198f
        helping relationships (change process
            objective), 194
        implementation, 195
        session steps, 195–196
        session summary, 195
        session tasks, 197
    14 needs clarification, 13
        handout/Needs Assessment, 200, 203

        handout/Resource Guide, 201, 204–205
        implementation, 200
        session steps, 200–201
        session summary, 199–200
        session tasks, 200–201
        social liberation (change process objective),
            199
    15 review and termination
        handout/Review, 207, 210
        implementation, 207
        self-efficacy and reinforcement manage-
            ment (change process objectives), 206
        session steps, 207–208
        session summary, 207
        session tasks, 208–209
AA
    "sobriety chips" as reinforcers, 15
    as social support resource, 195
Addiction treatment (Great Britain), and TTM,
    2
Alcohol Abstinence Self-Efficacy Scale, 20
Alcohol Effects Questionnaire, 71
Alcohol Expectancy Questionnaire, 71
Alcohol Use Disorders Identification Test
    (AUDIT), 52, 56f–58f
Assertion training, 23–24
Assessment methods
    clinical interview, 30–31
    Readiness Ruler, 29–30, 30f
    University of Rhode Island Change Assess-
        ment Scale, 31

Brown, Dr. Sandy, 71

Centers for Disease Control and Prevention,
    and TTM, 2
Change, 7, *see also* Processes of change
    success factors, 10
Cognitive techniques, *see also* Framing
    cognitive recognition, 24
        in contemplation stage, 12
        in precontemplation stage, 11
    cognitive restructuring, 24
        in action stage, 12
Communication
    effective, 155
    passive/aggressive/assertive, 152–153
Conditioning, *see* Linkages of later stage
    processes
Contemplation, *see* Stages of change
Cravings, 173, *see also* Urges
Crossover, *see* Decision balancing

Decisional balance, 9–10, 11, 12, 84
    "crossover" (in contemplation stage), 12, 85
Dissonance concept, 81

Environmental restructuring, 24
    in action stage, 12

Framing, in preparation stage, 12

Goal setting, 23
    in preparation stage, 12
Group sessions on substance abuse, *see also*
        Group work refresher
    early stages of change, 3, *see also* P/C/P
        sessions
    facilitator requirements, 28, 34
    group rules, 41, 128–129
    group size, 29
    intake screening and assessment, 29–31
        group assignments, 31–32
        multiple stages of change/types of
            substances per client, 31
    later (action-oriented) stages of change, 3, *see
        also* A/M sessions
    session format
        change process objective, 32
        content objectives, 33
        implementation, 33
        materials, 33
        rationale, 32–33
        step-by-step session tasks, 33
        summary, 33
    session frequency and length, 29
    session targets, 3
    setting, 28–29
    termination process, 208
    treatment overview, 27–28
Group work refresher, 33
    group facilitation techniques, 34–35
    leading groups, 33–34

Handouts
    A/M sessions, 126
        Alternatives to Using, 181
        Effective Communication, 155
        Maladaptive Thoughts, 171
        Managing Criticism, 165
        Meditation, 145
        My Action Plan, 188
        Needs Assessment, 203
        Practicing Refusals, 160
        Resource Guide, 204–205

    Review (session 11), 186–187
    Review (session 15), 210
    Rewarding My Success, 150
    Stages of Change, 133f
    To Manage Cravings and Urges I Can . . .,
        176
    What Can I Do After a Slip?, 193
    When Am I the Most Tempted to Use?,
        139
    Where Am I?, 134
P/C/P sessions, 38
    A Day in the Life, 51
    Alcohol Use Disorders Identification Test
        (AUDIT), 56
    AUDIT–What Does It Mean?, 58
    "Carolyn's Pros and Cons for Alcohol
        Use," 89f
    Choosing a Solution: "Dave's Options,"
        112f
    Drug Screening Inventory, 66
    Goal Setting and Change Plan (Example),
        117f
    My Expectations about Substance Use, 74
    My Goal Setting and Change Plan, 118
    My Pros and Cons for Substance Use,
        90
    My Relationships, 95
    My Relationships (Example), 96
    Problem-Solving Examples, 111f
    Review, 124
    Scoring the AUDIT, 57
    Scoring the Drug Screening Inventory, 67
    Stages of Change, 45f
    The Hardest Times for Me Are . . ., 107
    The Most Tempting Times for Me Are . . .,
        106
    What Can Alcohol Do?, 59–60
    What Can Drugs Do?, 68–69
    What Hats Do I Wear?, 101f
    What I Value Most in Life, 83
    Where Am I?, 46f
    Who is Concerned?, 79

Intervention, *see* Group sessions on substance
    abuse

Linkages of later stage processes
    concurrent functioning of stimulus control,
        counterconditioning, and reinforcement
        management, 14–16, 15f
        and Skinner's theory, 15
        and Pavlov's theory, 14

Maladaptive thoughts, 171
Motivation
    dynamic state vs. trait conceptualization, 1
    motivational approach introduction to clients,
        40–41
    motivational strategies, 20–21
Motivational interviewing (MI)/MI style, 17–18
    preparation for change goal, 19
    principles
        avoid argumentation, 18
        develop discrepancy, 18
        express empathy, 18
        roll with resistance, 18
        support self-efficacy, 19
    and resistance, 19–20
    and TTM framework, 20

National Cancer Institute, and TTM, 2
National Heart, Lung, and Blood Institute, and
    TTM, 2
National Institute on Alcohol Abuse and Alco-
    holism
    and information on physiological effects of
        alcohol, 53
    and TTM, 2
National Institute on Drug Abuse, and TTM,
    2
Needs clarification, 25
    in maintenance stage, 13
Negative thoughts, see Maladaptive thoughts

P/C/P sessions, 3
    1 psychoeducation, 11
        consciousness raising (change process
            objective), 39
        handout/Stages of Change, 41, 45f
        handout/Where Am I?, 43, 46f
        implementation, 40
        session steps, 40–43
        session summary, 40
        tasks, 43–44
    2 Timeline Followback, 11
        consciousness raising (change process
            objective), 47
        handout/A Day in the Life, 48–49, 51
        implementation, 48
        session steps, 48–49
        session summary, 47–48
        session task, 49–50
    3 psychoeducation, 11, 20
        consciousness raising (change process
            objective), 52

        handout/Alcohol Use Disorders Identifica-
            tion Test (AUDIT), 53, 54, 56f
        handout/AUDIT–What Does It Mean?, 54,
            58
        handout/Scoring the Audit, 54, 57
        handout/What Can Alcohol Do?, 54,
            59–60
        implementation, 53
        session steps, 53–54
        session summary, 53
        session tasks, 54–55
    4 psychoeducation, 11, 20
        consciousness raising (change process
            objective), 61
        handout/Drug Screening Inventory, 62–63,
            66
        handout/Scoring the Drug Screening
            Inventory, 63, 67
        handout/What Can Drugs Do?, 63, 68–
            69
        implementation, 62
        session steps, 62–63
        session summary, 62
        session tasks, 64–65
    5 cognitive recognition, 11
        consciousness raising (change process
            objective), 70
        handout/My Expectations About Substance
            Use, 71, 74
        implementation, 71
        session steps, 71–72
        session summary, 70–71
        session tasks, 72–73
    6 cognitive recognition, 11
        handout/Who Is Concerned?, 76, 79
        implementation, 76
        self-reevaluation/dramatic relief (change
            process objectives), 75
        session steps, 76–77
        session summary, 76
        session tasks, 77–78
    7 values clarification, 12
        handout/What I Value Most in Life, 81, 83
        implementation, 81
        self-reevaluation (change process objective),
            80
        session steps, 81–82
        session summary, 80
        session tasks, 82
    8 decision making, 12
        decisional balance (change process objec-
            tive), 84

handout/Carolyn's Pros and Cons for
   Alcohol Use, 86, 89f
handout/My Pros and Cons for Alcohol
   Use, 86, 90
implementation, 85
session steps, 85–87
session summary, 84–85
session tasks, 87–88
9 cognitive recognition, 12
environmental reevaluation (change
   process objective), 91
handout/My Relationships, 92, 95
handout/My Relationships (Example), 93,
   96
implementation, 92
session steps, 92–93
session summary, 92
session tasks, 93–94
10 role clarification, 12
environmental reevaluation (change
   process objective), 97
handout/What Hats Do I Wear?, 98, 101f
implementation, 98
session steps, 98–99
session summary, 97
session tasks, 99–100
11 self-test for temptation/confidence and
   problem solving, 11, 12, 20
handout/The Hardest Times for Me
   Are . . . , 103, 107
handout/The Most Tempting Times for Me
   Are . . . , 103, 106
implementation, 103
self-efficacy (change process objective), 102
session steps, 103–105
session summary, 102
session tasks, 104–106
12 problem solving, 12
handout/Choosing A Solution: "Dave's
   Options," 109–110, 112f
handout/Problem Solving Examples, 109,
   111f
implementation, 109
self-efficacy (change process objective), 108
session steps, 109–110
session summary, 108
session tasks, 110
13 goal setting, 12
handout/Goal Setting and Change Plan
   (Example), 115, 117f
handout/My Goal Setting and Change
   Plan, 115, 118

implementation, 114
self-liberation (change process objective),
   113
session steps, 114–115
session summary, 113–114
session tasks, 116
14 review and termination
handout/Review, 120, 124
implementation, 120
rationale and objectives, 119
session steps, 120–121
session summary, 119
session tasks, 121–122
Pavlov, Ivan, 14
Precontemplation, *see* Stages of change
Preparation, *see* Stages of change
Problem solving, 22–23
in preparation stage, 12
Processes of change, 8
behavioral processes
   counterconditioning, 8–9, 12, 13, 140, 151,
      156, 161, 166, 172, 177
   helping relationships, 9, 12, 13, 194,
      195
   reinforcement management, 9, 12, 13, 146,
      151, 156, 161, 166, 172, 177, 206
   self-liberation, 9, 12, 13, 113, 182,
      189
   stimulus control, 8, 12, 13, 135, 166, 172,
      177
experiential processes
   consciousness raising, 8, 11, 13–14, 39, 47,
      52, 61, 70, 127
   dramatic relief, 8, 11, 75
   environmental reevaluation, 8, 11, 12, 14,
      91, 97
   self-reevaluation, 8, 11, 12, 14, 75, 80
   social liberation, 8, 12, 13, 14, 199
as facilitators, 1, *see also* Linkages of later
   stage processes
   early stage processes/level of awareness,
      13–14
   later stage processes, 14–16
peaks, 9
and stages, 9, 10t
and techniques, 16
Professional contacts/suggested resources
references, 211a–212a
training information, 212a
websites, 212a
Psychoeducation, 21
and precontemplation stage, 11

Reflective listening, 81
Reinforcement, 25, *see also* Linkages of later
    stage processes
  in action stage, 12
Relapse
  high-risk situations for "slips," 162
  prevention strategies, 1-2, 23
    planning in action stage, 12
  and recycling, 10, 13, 190-191
Relaxation techniques, 23
  in action stage, 12
Research opportunities, 3
Resistance
  and MI, 19-20
  and working with clients "where they are," 35
Robert Wood Johnson Foundation, and TTM, 2
Rohsenow, Dr. Damaris, 71
Role clarification, 25
Role play, 24
  in action stage, 12
Rollnick, Dr. Stephen, 48

Self-efficacy, 10, 12, 13, 102, 108, 206
Skinner, B. F., 15, 25
Sobell, Drs. Linda and Mark, 48
Social cognitive theory (Bandura), influence on
    TTM, 10
Social and communication skills enhancement,
    25
  in maintenance stage, 13
Stages of change (P/C/P/A/M), 7, 11
  precontemplation, 7, 11
    and MI, 19
    placement in group setting, 32
  contemplation, 7, 11-12
    and "crossover," 85
  preparation, 7, 12
  action, 7, 12
  maintenance, 7, 13
  cycling/recycling and success, 10, 13, 190
  introduction, 41
    "staging exercise," 42-43, 207
    "Where Am I?" handout, 43, 46f
  and processes, 9, 10t

Techniques, 16, 21, 22t
  assertion training, 23-24, 102-107
  assessment and feedback, 25-26, 52-60,
    61-69
  cognitive recognition, 11, 12, 24, 166-171
  cognitive restructuring, 12, 24, 172-176
  decision making, 12, 84-90
  environmental restructuring, 12, 24, 91-96
  framing, 12, 24, 189-193
  goal setting, 12, 23, 113-118
  needs clarification, 13, 25, 102-107, 199-
    205
  problem solving/brainstorming, 12, 22-23,
    108-112, 177-181
  and processes of change, 16, 39-46
  psychoeducation, 11, 21, 161-165, 166-172
  reinforcement, 12, 25, 146-150, 156-160,
    161-165
  relapse prevention planning, 12, 182-188
  relaxation, 12, 23, 140-145
  role clarification, 12, 25, 97-101
  role play, 24, 158-160
  social and communication skills enhance-
    ment, 13, 25, 151-155, 194-198
  the Timeline Followback, 11, 47-51
  values clarification, 12, 21-22, 75-79, 80-83
Timeline Followback (TLFB), 26, 48
  in precontemplation stage, 11
Transtheoretical model (TTM) of behavior
    change, 1, 7-9, *see also* Process of change;
    Stages of change
  uses (multiple interventions/populations), 2
Treatment, *see* Group sessions on substance
    abuse
Trigger
  categories, 103, 107
  identification, 103, 135-139
  and unhealthy thoughts, 173
12-step groups, as social support resource, 195

Urges, 173, *see also* Cravings

Values clarification, 21
  in contemplation stage, 12